Historical Explorations in Medicine and Psychiatry

HERTHA RIESE, M.D., was born in Berlin and studied medicine at the University of Berlin. After her marriage to Dr. Walther Riese, she finished her last semester at the newly established University of Frankfurt am Main, the second woman to be registered for admission to the academic career. She studied psychiatry at that university and was soon assigned to the service of Dr. Walther Riese, whose laboratory for comparative neurology and neuropathology at the Parc Zoologique de Vincennes was associated with the Sorbonne.

While living in Europe, Hertha Riese was the director of a family counseling clinic affiliated with the International Association for the Protection of Motherhood, an early feminist organization; a counselor at the Lycée de Jeunes Filles de Lyon, Versailles, and Vincennes; and a teacher at the Catholic School of Social Work. In the United States, she was cofounder (with Kitty Dennis) and director for twenty years of the Educational Therapy Center in Richmond, Virginia, established to combat the emotional and educational consequences of racial discrimination.

Since her retirement, Dr. Riese has been the consultant and treating psychiatrist to a number of agencies. She coedited (with Walther Riese) a series of sociopsychiatric books and she has published numerous articles and three books, most recently *Heal the Hurt Child*. Dr. Riese has been invited by many nations to deliver papers, has received numerous awards for achievement, and holds an honorary doctorate degree in law from Virginia State College.

Historical Explorations
in Medicine and Psychiatry

Hertha Riese, Editor

with 20 contributors

Springer Publishing Company

New York

Springer Publishing Company, Inc.
200 Park Avenue South
New York, N.Y. 10003

78   79   80   81   82   /   10   9   8   7   6   5   4   3   2   1

Library of Congress Cataloging in Publication Data

Main entry under title:

Historical explorations in medicine and psychiatry.

    Festschrift in honor of W. Riese.
    Bibliography: p.
    1. Psychiatry—History—Addresses, essays, lectures. 2. Medicine—
History—Addresses, essays, lectures. 3. Riese, Walther, 1890–1976.
I. Riese, Hertha Pataky, 1892–   II. Riese, Walther, 1890–1976.
[DNLM: 1. History of medicine. 2. Psychiatry—History. 3. Historiography.
WM11.1 H672]
RC438.H54   616.8'9   78–17231
ISBN 0–8261–2290–6
ISBN 0–8261–2291–4 pbk.

Printed in the United States of America

616.89

H62

79531

To the memory of

Dr. Walther Riese

Contents

Preface

This book is the outgrowth of the mutual friendship and community of minds of Walther Riese and a number of his friends. The volume reflects the variety of those interests and achievements which associated Walther Riese with attuned thinkers and researchers—kinfolk in the humanitarianism of his historical view of neurology and psychiatry.

Through reflection, which is the objectivation of his vegetating self, the human creature becomes the author of the human being, or man. Reflection implies conceiving or registering existence through the "word." Reflection presupposes the awareness of what has gone by and the telling of it, or the relating of what precedes to what follows, or the comparison of changes in quantification and qualification. As a result, being becomes an historical event, a registered datum of history.

All of us are and must be Aeneas. He remembered that in his growing days he was carried on his father's shoulders; in turn, he felt impelled to carry his father lovingly on his shoulders to save him from death in the destruction of Troy. The loving reverence of the past and its contribution kept Aeneas undefeated in spirit. As the son of a culture, he brought along the building blocks for Rome, a Rome that did not remain a legend but became a tribute to mankind's indebtedness to the temporally and spatially remote past. This indebtedness causes us, in turn, to transmit our search for knowledge and self-recognition to the next generation. Thus, we provide our descendants with an ever more elevated point of vantage and with ever greater discrimination. Ultimately, theirs will be an understanding of man himself—of the totality of his becoming.

This continual process of unfolding is represented by this book. It begins with the discussion of the historical method and shows in specific instances how, through time, man registers and interprets his developing knowledge and skills and thus reaps benefits of learning, thought, and action from the study of history. In doing so, he not only learns from the past but endows it and, carrying it on his shoulders, transmits a new reality to be further endowed. The book begins, as it should, with what precedes—the ancient. It ends with the modern and a bold outlook on the future gained by the descent of acute thinkers into the mines of the recent past.

Though all chapters of the book grow from common roots, they also form a closed continuum, for the endowment of man has no beginning and no end. In each section of the book, one or more chapters emphasize how the style of a historical period depended on the previous specific discoveries or the evolution of views—that is, on the accruing steps in understanding the past as a teacher. Other chapters show the present revealing the meaning (not merely the events) of the past and fathering a clearly and boldly envisioned future.

Acknowledgments

Dr. Carlo Castellani first solicited the contributions to this book. Mrs. Louis Morton, retired research librarian of the Medical College of Virginia, translated the articles originally written in French. After the sudden and unexpected death of Mrs. Frances Benedek, Walther Riese's polyglot secretary of over 25 years, Mrs. Peggy Rothweiler, my secretary, performed the enormous task of typing and correspondence in addition to her already full schedule.

Acknowledgment is owed to Dr. Kenneth Newell for a last review and condensation of my editorial text, to Drs. Eric Deudon, Richard Laurent, and Roland Villars, M.T.S., for similar aid in reference to the original French and English texts, and to Drs. Alan Entin and Humberto Gomez for coming to my aid in reading or verifying the text at a critical moment when Walther Riese's terminal illness and his death coincided with the publication deadline. Acknowledgment also is due to Mr. Melvin Shaffer, associate professor at the Medical College of Virginia and director of the Visual Education Department of the college and to his associate staff member, Mr. James Anderson, for much appreciated help in their field.

H. R.

Contributors

PROFESSOR HENRI BARUK was the reorganizer and director from 1931 to 1968 of the National Psychiatric Hospital of Charenton which was made famous by Esquirol. He was the founder of the first laboratory of experimental psychiatry of France, where he produced catatonia in apes by the use of bulbocapnine, the neurotropic bacterium coli, with bile, ACTH, etc. He is director of the Ecole des Hautes Etudes of the Sorbonne, professor at the Medical College of Paris, and member of the French Academy of Medicine. To the Rockefeller Foundation is due the credit of having subventioned Dr. Baruk's studies under the great Dutch scientists Kappers, Brower, and De Jung, and later the foundation of the laboratory at Charenton. Baruk's experimental studies of toxic action led to the discovery of the dangers of cardiazol on the psychism. Surgical and other experiments revealed the dangers of electroshock and lobotomy. Professor Baruk initiated a successful international campaign to prevent their use. Experimental studies on animals of the actions of hormones on the brain found their application in man (the hyperfolliative psychoses). Professor Baruk's view that a "destructive prognosis" for schizophrenia was unjustified because its causes and cures could be found was internationally acclaimed. Professor Baruk is the founder of the Society Moreau de Tours and the editor of its journal, which is in honor of the first psychiatrist to have seen the action of toxic substances on the brain and the importance of oneirism. He has published 22 books and 300 articles in the areas of these studies as well as on moral consciousness in the wake of the experience of the Hitler period.

JEANNE L. BRAND, PH.D., is chief of the International Programs Division, Extramural Programs, National Library of Medicine. She is a member of numerous American and foreign professional societies for the history of medicine. In addition to more than 20 articles, she has authored *Doctors and the State: The British Medical Profession and Government Action in Public Health, 1870–1912* (1965) and, with Dr. George Mora, coedited *Psychiatry and Its History* (1970).

FRANÇOISE DUFAY, M.D., has been on the staff of the neurological and psychiatric clinic of the university hospital in Besançon since 1967. She studied medicine in Besançon and Strasbourg, and her areas of psychiatric specialization include relaxation and speech pathology.

H. F. ELLENBERGER, M.D., taught psychiatry in the Menninger School of Psychiatry and McGill University in Montreal. Since 1962, he has been professor of Criminology at the University of Montreal. In 1970, the German Criminological Association awarded him the Beccaria Prize. He is the author of about 160 articles and encyclopedia entries in psychiatry, psychology, and criminology. His main work, which has been translated into French, German, Italian, Japanese, and Spanish, is the *Discovery of the Unconscious* (1970).

HENRI EY, M.D., is former chairman of the Department of Psychiatry at the Medical College of Paris; head physician at the Psychiatric Hospital, Bonneval; and chief editor for the psychiatry section of the Encyclopédie médico-chirurgicale. His main publications are three psychiatric studies: *The Conscience* (1963, 1968), translated into German, Spanish, and Japanese; *Treatise on Hallucinations* (1973); and *Hughlings Jackson's Theories: A Departure for an Organo-dynamic Model in Psychiatry* (in press). His *Textbook of Psychiatry*, written with P. Bernand and Ch. Brisset and translated into Spanish and Italian, is in its fifth edition.

ERNST FISCHER, M.D., a neuromuscular physiologist, is professor emeritus of Physiology at Virginia Commonwealth University.

IAGO GALDSTON, M.D., turned from the field of internal medicine and public health to psychiatry because of his long-standing interest in the psychological component of illness. At that period he also turned to the history of medicine. He has an extensive array of publications in all these fields to his credit, most recently: *Medicine in Transition* and *Psychiatry and the Human Condition*. He has taught at New York University, Fordham, and the New York Medical College. Dr. Galdston, who was the founder and first president of the American Association of Directors of Psychiatric Residency Training, has served as secretary for both the American Association of Medical History and the New York Academy of Medicine and as consultant to the Grant Division on Medical History of the National Institute of Mental Health. In 1972, Dr. Galdston was awarded the Gold Medal of the American College of Psychiatrists for "significant achievement, contributions, and leadership in the field of psychiatry."

WILLIAM GOODDY, M.D., is fellow of University College, London; fellow of the Royal College of Physicians of London; and consulting neurologist to the Royal Navy. He is senior physician, the National Hospital for Nervous Diseases, Queen Square, London; consultant neurologist, University College Hospital, St. Richard's Hospital, Chichester, King Edward VII Hospital, Midhurst; honorary neurologist, the Italian Hospital, London. Dr. Gooddy is also president-elect, Association of British Neurologists, and honorary member of Neurological Associations of France and Australia. He has written numerous publications about time and the nervous system.

PROFESSOR PAUL W. HARKINS is the author of *St. John Chrysostom: Baptismal Discourses* (1963) and *Galen: On the Passions and Errors of the Soul,* coauthored with Dr. Walther Riese (1963). Another volume, *The Polemics of Chrysostom,* is in press, and the book *Chrysostom's Apologetics* is in preparation. After a long career of teaching classical languages and philosophy, Professor Harkins retired in 1975 from Xavier University, Cincinnati, Ohio, where he was professor emeritus of Classical Languages, and plans to translate Chrysostom's vast scriptural commentaries.

SAUL JARCHO, M.D., a practicing internist, is editor-in-chief of the *Bulletin of the New York Academy of Medicine.* He has been consultant to the Grant Division on Medical History of the National Institute of Mental Health and president of the American Association for the History of Medicine.

PROFESSOR F. LHERMITTE is chairman of the Department of Neurology and Neuropsychology at the Hôpital de la Salpêtrière, Paris, and director of Neurological Research at the National Institute of Health and Medical Research, National Center for Scientific Research, Paris. Professor Lhermitte has published over 300 articles dealing primarily with multiple sclerosis, demyelinating diseases, cerebrovascular disturbances, and of course, neuropsychology.

GEORGE MORA, M.D., is research associate in the Department of the History of Science and Medicine, Yale University, and medical director of the Astor Home and Clinics for Children, Rhinebeck, New

York. He is also on the faculty of the medical schools of Columbia University; Union University, Albany; and the New York Medical College. He has written extensively on the history of psychiatry, and is coeditor with Jeanne L. Brand of *Psychiatry and Its History* (1970).

MARGARET REINHOLD, M.D., member of the Royal College of Physicians of London, is a consulting psychiatrist who has published numerous works on neurological and psychiatric subjects.

M. SCHACHTER, M.D., has been head consulting physician in Child Neuropsychiatry of the Marseille Society of Childhood Deficiency (1945-1975), assistant professor of pediatric neuropsychiatry at the Medical College of Marseille; fellow of the Royal Society of Medicine of London, active member of the French Pediatric Society of Neuropsychology, correspondent to the Medico-Psychological Society of France, active member of the French Society of the History of Medicine and of the French Society of Psychology, and correspondent member of the German Society for Childhood and Youth Psychiatry. Dr. Schachter has published on the problem of underweight, Mongolism, the child that has become delinquent, the enuretic child. He is coauthor of four books and numerous articles on similar subjects, on embryonic and child encephalopathies, on comparison of the Rorschach test in childhood and adulthood, and on drawing tests, in particular the Wartegg test.

PIERRE MAXIME SCHUHL is a member of the Institut de France, director of the *Revue Philosophique*, Dr. honoris causa of the University of Rome, and honorable professor at the Sorbonne. He is the author of some twenty philosophical works on Plato, imagination and realization, imagination and the marvelous, the format of Greek thought, and three essays on Montaigne.

RUDOLPH E. SIEGEL (1900–1975) received his medical degree in 1923 from Göttingen, Germany. In 1938, Dr. Siegel settled in Buffalo, where he practiced medicine, specializing in cardiovascular disease. At the time of his death he was associate clinical professor emeritus, State University of New York in Buffalo. In March, 1975, the School of Medicine and the Medical Historical Society of Buffalo joined in honoring Dr. Siegel "in recognition of his distinguished contributions to the history of medicine." Dr. Siegel was the author of many articles on his experimental work in physiology and medicine; he also published over thirty-five articles on the history of medicine as well as four volumes on Galen: *Galen's System of Physiology and Medicine* (1968),

Galen on Sense Perception (1970), *Galen on Psychology, Psychopathology and Function and Diseases of the Nervous System* (1973), *Galen on the Affected Parts* (1976).

JEAN-LOUIS SIGNORET, M.D., is professeur agrégé on the faculty of medicine of the Hôpital de Salpêtrière, Paris.

HANS SYZ, M.D., came to the United States in 1921 and served on the staffs of the Henry Phipps Psychiatric Clinic of the Johns Hopkins Hospital, Baltimore, Maryland; the New York State Psychiatric Institute; and the New York Hospital–Cornell Medical College. He has published in the fields of animal experimentation, experimental psychology, and clinical problems and group dynamics. Among his numerous publications are journal articles and encyclopedia entries on group- or phyloanalysis and phylopathology. Dr. Syz is associated with The Lifwynn Foundation, Westport, Connecticut, an organization devoted to research in human behavior.

ILZA VEITH, PH.D., is professor and vice-chairman, Department of the History of Health Sciences, and professor, Department of Psychiatry, University of California, San Francisco. She has also served as consultant to the Grant Division on Medical History of the National Institute of Mental Health.

PROFESSOR ROBERT VOLMAT is head of the Clinique Neurologique et Psychiatrique, Centre Hospitalier Regional, Besançon. He is the founder and president of the Comité d'Honneur de la Société Internationale de Psychopathologie de L'Expression, Besançon.

Prologue:
In Memory of Walther Riese—
Author, Physician, Teacher, Man

This book was originally meant to be an homage to Dr. Walther Riese on his eighty-fifth birthday, June 30, 1975, offered by a number of his distinguished friends. Since "books have their fate," this book has become a memorial to him. We are deprived of the privilege of having him with us to be honored for his endowment to the future that he keenly had in mind even during those years when he had to turn his scholarship almost exclusively to the study of history and thought in medicine.

The number and scope of Walther Riese's publications is vast. Due to his remarkable eloquence and style in three languages, he could publish for a large and significant audience. His 15 books and 277 articles encompass neurology, neuroanatomy, comparative neurology, neuropathology, medical psychology (forensic psychology, pathography, psychiatry), history of medicine, and philosophy of medicine. Only recently, *Conception of Disease* appeared in Italian, translated by Dr. Guiseppe Ongaro.* His collected publications on aphasia, edited by Professor Yvan Lebrun and Dr. Richard Hoops, have just been published.**

Many of these publications are recognized as classics, among them: *Principles of Neurology in the Light of History and Their Present Use, La pensée causale en médecine, La pensée morale en médecine: premiers principes d'une éthique médicale, The Conception of*

---

*Milan: Episteme Editrice, 1975.
**Muncie, Ind.: Ball State University, and Amsterdam: Swets and Zeitlinger, 1977.

Disease: Its History, Its Versions and Its Nature, and *A History of Neurology.* Others, like his psychopathological studies and books on Van Gogh and the Austrian poet Georg Trakl, were pioneers of their kind, and his medicolegal books and other publications were quoted as guidelines by the Supreme Courts of Weimar Germany and Switzerland.

In all areas of his endeavors, Walther Riese made an original contribution. His neuroanatomic studies were never merely descriptive. His early interest was the problem of the relationship of the parts to the whole, which he verified in his comparative neurological studies of various species, in his clinical studies, and his studies on malformations. This approach proved very fruitful in his studies of the brains of men of genius. It ultimately led to his preoccupation with the problem of integration. His studies of the shape of body and brain of the aquatic mammals reflected his concern with problems of adaptation to the environment; his studies of hibernating mammals dealt with the reversible modification of the nerve cell and the endocrinological substratum in reference to the active and dormant stages.

Of highest interest was his comparative neurological research on the marsupials, the brown bear, and other new-born mammals, the investigations of which were devoted to the sustained (natural) and not the experimentally provoked behavior. Behavior was being *observed.* The marsupials in their earliest stages of life in the pouch are extremely small-sized, immature structures that nevertheless display active, complex, and appropriate behavior. The cubs of the huge-sized brown bear are of miniature size. With a cell structure and organization that is not even outlined, they perform the spontaneous and adapted behavior of the new-born mammal. Riese observed closely the animal's progressive behavior and, regardless of the degree of development, he studied their central nervous system or brain structure at closely spaced, consequential phases of development. The organism was presumed to function as an integrated whole. At no stage, therefore, was developmental behavior related to isolated structural elements in disregard of others. Attention had to be and was centered not only on the first appearance of certain finished structural fragments, presumably responsible for the behavior displayed by the embryo, but also on still immature structures to which nobody can deny some type of function and cooperation in behavior. In a number of species and orders no parallelism between nervous behavior and nervous structures was found. Animals born with an undeveloped cell structure and organization were found to be capable of purposeful behavior on a level not to be expected at such immature stages of structural development. In some instances where behavioral maturation preceded structural maturation, the latter development after birth was observed to be remarkably fast. *Functional development predates structural development and contributes to the realization of its potentials.*

In clinical neurology, Walther Riese was among the pioneers in research on tonus in its physiological and pathological aspects, mind blindness, aphasia, cerebral localization, and the phantom limb. His thorough knowledge of the anatomy, physiology, and pathology of the central nervous system made him a splendid diagnostician as well as theoretician, and placed him in the forefront of forensic psychiatry and neurology.

A socially responsible person, he used his magistral diagnostic marksmanship on behalf of brain injured veterans and the brain injured victims of accidents, in particular those injured at work. These experiences, combined with his year-long studies of the aged, the aphasic, and those affected by tumors of the central nervous system— followed by the postmortem study of the affected central nervous organ of the individuals he had observed so thoroughly during their illness—were reflected ultimately in a masterly integration of knowledge in his *Principles of Neurology,* with its two key chapters "Vulnerability" and "Diaschisis." The concept of vulnerability supplants the concept of localization. The brain, even the organism, functions always as a whole. *Function* cannot be localized in any specific area of the brain. The substratum does not give evidence of any specific function, nor can specific function be elicited experimentally from any specific area. Electric stimulation of the so-called speech center does not elicit speech. Only *symptoms* can be referred to injured tissue; symptoms disclose clearly that a specific function is vulnerable at the injured area. The concept of diaschisis, shock, or action at a distance is evidence of the fact that the brain functions always as a whole. This concept is the clue to the formerly unsolved riddle of why symptoms would appear where, according to theory, they were not to be expected (as for instance, speech disorders when the right hemisphere is affected in the right-handed person), or why some symptoms are transitory and others persist. The concept warrants avoidance of erroneous localization of the affection and permits early prognostication of the ultimate outcome. Even his thoughts and experiences on the therapy of the aphasics benefited by the experience gained, for instance, in the study of the newborn and infant brain at various phases of its early development and the realization that the *function* does not, as assumed to that time, presume *structure* but that *function and structure reciprocally presume one another. Function realizes its own potentially outlined opportunity.*

This finding was confirmed in his study of the brains of aged
scholars of extraordinary stature, such as Ludwig Edinger, von Monakow, and Trigant Burrow, who had proceeded to the end with their
inquiries and had retained a highly preserved cellullar structure and
stratification. In aphasics, he discovered preserved functions despite
the tissue destruction expected to warrant it. *Function outlived its
injured substratum.* As Walther Riese worded it, *The most important
attainments in early childhood are made with an immature brain. The
most important attainments in advanced age are made with a dis-
integrating brain.*°

This finding has therapeutic, rehabilitational, sociomedical, social,
and racial implications. For instance, Walther Riese emphatically insisted on keeping human—not just scheduled therapeutical—contact
with the aphasic: on speaking with him, keeping his sense of dignity
alive, and making him feel that he is not left out, thereby soliciting
emotionally sustained speech function that will recruit and restore its
anatomic substratum or "organ of speech." Similarly, mental capacities
of the indigent and racial potentials cannot be fairly assessed unless
full, prolonged opportunity is given to build up a substratum withered
under environmental disadvantage, whether climatic, socioeconomic,
or psychological in nature.

Dr. Walther Riese was well served by a logical and methodical
acuity of the highest order, qualities exercised from high-school time
on by the thorough study of philosophy, the history of thought, and
finally, the history of medical thought. The French Kantian philosopher, Lachieze Rey, considered Walther Riese the greatest and
clearest interpreter of Kant's philosophy. In admiration of the depth
and conciseness of his writing, he wrote: "*Chaque phrase une doctrine.*" In Kant's philosophy, Dr. Riese found the philosophical foundation for the reciprocity, rather than the one way dependence, of function from its anatomical substratum; in the study of history, he found
the greatness of predecessors. In recent years, he renewed our awareness that the historical concept of sympathy in Brown-Sequard's original formulation—the action at a distance—deserved to be unearthed
and brought to fruition.

Walther Riese's concept of history is not one of periods unfolding one after another but of all stages of development coexisting at
all times. Not only is the past the teacher of all descendent generations, but each new generation from its point of vantage finds its un-

---

°*The Principles of Neurology in the Light of History and Their Present Use*
(Baltimore: Williams and Wilkins, 1950).

derstanding of historical events. Through new interpretation it modifies the past.

We cannot end without referring to Dr. Riese's important studies on methodology, observation, experimentation, his studies on Claude Bernard, and above all, his book *La pensée causale en médecine*.

Walther Riese has been honored greatly; he received unusually prolonged support for research by the Rockefeller Foundation, the Grant Division of the Department of Health, Education, and Welfare, and the analogous French Government Research Division. He was a consultant to DHEW and consultant neuropathologist to the Virginia Mental Hygiene Department from 1941 until his retirement in 1960.

There are many who remember him as a teacher of unique impact. "Sympathy" and reciprocity prevailed between students and teacher. In fact, although Walther Riese enjoyed the friendship of men great in their field, sterling in character, and genuine in love, he felt inspired by the joyful and enthusiastic attention of his students, who, in particular during the last 20 years of his academic career, when great territorial distances, oceans, and death separated him from proven friends, kept the glow of life kindled in him.

—Hertha Riese

Part I

Historiography, Methodology, and Classification

History requires no justification; instead, it justifies man as a supra-biological creature that seeks a continuous meaning in his experiences. Thereby he immortalizes them and establishes mankind as the creation of the reflecting consciousness of both the individual and mankind. One essay in this section contains a variety of suggestions on how to write history that is truly an enlightening testimony to the continuity of his consciousness (Brand). The other essays explain how any significant discovery and its occurrence at a specific period are embedded in the productive and receptive terrain of the total civilization (Siegel and Fischer). Siegel also refers to Walther Riese's idea that the endowment provided by history is not one-directional. With every new meaning that the maturing cultures applies to the facts of the past, more of the extant historical source material becomes inspiring, and the student transmits it to a student in an even more remote future. This continual reciprocity of endowment insures that the consciousness of the individual and that of the universal remain identical.

According to Siegel, the study of history is justified because the fundamental processes of thought do not change. Antiquity and a more recent period can discourse; they may disagree, but their grammar is the same. Siegel is aware of changing concepts and interpretations that provide the substance of the discourse, for example, concepts of matter. New discoveries may shed light on tentative explanations in the past and thereby provide answers to questions left open for centuries. Siegel traces some changing concepts through the ages. For example, the idea of the circulation of blood was based on Hippocrates' ideas and was significantly advanced by Galen's philosophical conjectures

1

and Harvey's experiments, but the idea became fully established as a fact only with Malpighi's demonstration of the capillaries through a microscope. Siegel's examples give concrete evidence how, through the ages, discoveries of clues led to closure of baffling gaps until the embedded final clue was uncovered by a breakthrough in the ripened culture or in the scientific or technological knowledge of the period. He writes, "One of the most attractive aspects of historiography is the demonstration of the evolution of ideas."

According to Siegel, the ancient thinkers and their discoveries should be recognized as precursors rather than slighted and consigned to oblivion. Their errors as well as insights are mines for enrichment and sources for the sorting of information and for the revaluation of concepts. The advancement of knowledge depends on the clarification reached by unbiased and respectful study of all periods, past and present.

In her essay, Brand also emphasizes integrity. Her study inevitably raises the question of the human equation in the interpretation of historical documents. She alludes, for instance, to the fact that the Enlightenment concept of man's rationality and consequently steady progress has been complemented by the modern concept of man's resilient irrationality. In the changed image of man, his highest achievements threaten to become the executors of his irrational nature. There the historian must be on guard that his work does not become the executor of his complexes and biases. So, too, do people on the historical scene; their personalities must be considered in establishing historical truth. Brand shows where the new sociological sciences and knowledge of the unconscious have served the study of history and where both a new endowment and limitations may be expected. She acknowledges a reciprocal enrichment: "Certainly both the professional historian and the professional psychiatrist have much to gain in the sharing of their experience."

Both Siegel and Brand are concerned about the judgmental attitude toward our forefathers and about the certitude with which some critics assign them merits and demerits. These critics disregard our forefathers' contributions that prove essential to the solution of long-standing problems. To consider the forefathers representative of only ephemeral periods implies that the critics consider themselves solely responsible for the stunning achievements of the present era and so either exclude themselves from the continuous chain of contributors who stand on their forefathers' shoulders or else consider modern wisdom as short-lived and futile as wisdom of earlier times. "Without an awareness of the far-reaching influences upon us from the past," says Siegel, "it would be difficult to teach any continuity in the history of ideas" or even, we might add, to remain human, to remember and foresee, to retain use of the tenses and, therefore, command of the "word."

Professor Fischer's essay leads us to the period of inductive thinking and into a changed new world. Up to the time of the Renaissance, man had to wait until nature revealed itself incidentally. He had, therefore, to be interested in knowledge for the sake of knowledge. As an expectant observer, he had to set aside his findings in the storeroom of human learning. Not until further fitting information was available could the scholar use it for an ever more satisfying complementation of findings, for example, the alleviation of human suffering and disease. Since Bacon discovered the laws of experimentation, man has learned to wrest from nature its secrets with a specific purpose in mind. He may proceed at a calculated risk with boldness or with a cautious scientific strategy that relies on an increasingly accurate body of knowledge, but he still cannot avoid trial and error. He has to retreat from unsuitable procedure and incorrect interpretations and speculate how to find a new line of attack. Fisher explains why, for instance, experimenters were deceived for a century by the assumption that they could prevent atrophy of denervated frog muscles by electric stimulation. They ignored the fact that the nerve had undergone a natural regeneration.

Fischer's essay reports many such errors of interpretation. They occurred because zealous experimentation over extended periods had not yet accumulated detailed knowledge about the function and interaction of nerves and muscles; their response to specific kinds of current; the intensity, frequency, and curve of flow of the current; etc. The purposefulness of the experimenter elicits such facts—sometimes to the limits of his capacity to assimilate them. He realizes their usefulness in achieving a specific aim and so can set a goal that is knowledge not only for its own sake (as it frequently used to be) but also for the sake of preventing or curing human suffering. In considering the far-reaching effects of the prolific aspects of the experimenter's work, we are reminded of the prologue on the theatre to Goethe's Faust and the director's statement, "*wer Vieles bringt, wird Manchem etwas bringen*" (He who brings a great deal has something to offer to many).

Jeanne L. Brand

1

The Historian
and the Psychiatrist:
Shared Understandings

One of America's best-known social historians, Arthur Schlesinger, Jr., observed that the historian of our times is usually "a professional, trained in his craft, a product of methodological discipline." The historian's vocation, Schlesinger continued, is a "quasi-priestly" one, "supposed to liberate him from the passions of the day, to assure him a serenity of perspective, and to consecrate him to the historian's classical ideal of objectivity."[1]

Most texts on historical method describe the historian's fundamental intellectual operation as a three-part task. He must first collect the probable sources of information. Next, he must subject them to critical examination and verification. Finally, drawing upon his own powers of analysis and with that desired "serenity of perspective," he attempts to reconstruct the past.[2]

In the last hundred years, the nature and number of the historian's sources of information have greatly expanded. Primary sources, or the testimony of contemporary eyewitnesses, constitute his foundation. To reconstruct an accurate version of reality, the historian must first locate, and then digest, a wide range of sources, extending from autobiographies, memoirs, diaries, speeches, memoranda kept by persons close to events, personal letters, official papers, contemporary surveys, newspaper accounts, textbooks, advertisements, and old maps to new aerial surveys. In recent years, new types of primary sources have

This paper is abridged from the author's chapter on "The Social Historian and the History of Psychiatry" in George Mora and Jeanne Brand, eds., *Psychiatry and Its History* (Springfield, Ill.: Charles C Thomas, c. 1970) by permission of the publisher.

4

swelled the possibilities: oral history transcriptions, dictating machine tapes, and motion pictures of sites or events. The historian may also develop his own history through interviews with persons having first-hand knowledge of the events he will describe. The medical and psychiatric historian may have the added responsibility of utilizing patient and hospital records, when they are available.

As one contemporary historian has observed: "The prevailing mood among professional historians nowadays is a chastened one in view of the immense mass of material and the infinite complexity of the phenomenon."[3]

A very real danger is that the historian may succumb to the fatal disease of pottering, lose himself in his sources, collect on and on, and never feel he has established a sufficiently solid base on which to build his analysis and narrative. Sir Charles Oman, the distinguished British historian, described a visit to Lord Acton's library after his death in 1902; Sir Charles saw the pigeonhole desks and cabinets with "literally thousands of compartments, into each of which were sorted little white slips" with topical references. One set was on early instances of a sympathetic feeling for animals, starting with Ulysses' old dog in Homer. Another was devoted to a collection of hard words about stepmothers in the national literature of many countries. Acton, for all his brilliance, wrote relatively little, and Sir Charles observed after his visit that "Acton had a great book hovering before his mind; what exactly it was I have never quite made out."[4]

Even while the historian is at work collecting source materials, he has entered into the second phase of his task: subjecting them to review in a careful process of internal and external criticism. He must at times determine authenticity of authorship, seek evidence of dates in unsigned, undated letters. The medieval historian, for example, knows that paper was rare in Europe before the fifteenth century and printing unknown, that there were no pencils before the sixteenth century or typewriters before the nineteenth. He has learned varieties of ink used in different periods and settings, and acquired a knowledge of paleography and diplomatics. He also knows that physical evidence can be, and has been, faked.

Facing the problem of meaning in his sources, the historian has familiarized himself with contemporary lexica. He also has acquired sufficient erudition about his period to know how to interpret the behavior of his characters in their contemporary setting.[5] Even when he has established the authenticity of a source, he must weigh the witness' credibility—his prejudices and his breadth of perspective.

The French economic historian, Marc Bloch, before his death in the French Resistance at the hands of the Nazis, had almost completed a delightful little book called *The Historian's Craft*. He observes that in weighing the credibility of a witness, the historian has to guard against not only the "forthright untruth" but the "embroidery of imaginary details upon the roughly trustworthy scheme of a narrative . . . for the purpose of embellishment." The historian must consider that "many witnesses deceive themselves in all good faith," "that the majority of minds are but mediocre recording cameras of the surrounding world," and that the observer's personal condition at the time and his degree of attention have an impact on the distortion of evidence, as does the possibility of outright error.[6]

In the end, after the historian decides which facts to reject and which to retain, he must fit them into the pattern he has developed. He knows that his data are incomplete and that he can only approximate reality. But he is buoyed by intellectual curiosity and a deep, almost sensuous, pleasure in making patterns out of fragments. In the process of imaginative reconstruction, he must make contact with the minds of those he is writing about; as R. G. Collingwood phrased it, he must re-enact the past in his own mind.[7]

But when he starts to build his pattern, he runs up against difficulties that his predecessors have struggled with—the problem of causality, for example. Does he believe that history is determined by impersonal forces, such as economic motivation? Does he see it fundamentally woven about great men and their individual roles in their time span?[8] Does he believe in, or deny, human progress? Does he see a plan of divine purpose or intervention, or think, as H. G. Wells put it, "that the inexorable laws of natural selection will result in the replacement of the present imperfect society by one in which a finer humanity will inhabit a more perfect world"?[9] Does he see societies as largely determined by their geographic and natural resources?

If the historian can recognize his own views on causality, can he, or should he, try to solve the problem of moral judgment in history? Does he feel with Herbert Butterfield that such judgments by historians are, very often, "pseudo-moral judgments, masquerading as moral ones, mixed and muddy affairs, part prejudice, part political animosity—with a dash of ethical flavouring wildly tossed into the concoction"—judgments pronounced by "impetuous adjudicators who have a rough idea of Henty heroes shining brightly against the background of something which is not quite cricket"?[10] Or, with Marc Bloch does he wonder: "Are we so sure of ourselves and our age as to divide the company of our forefathers into the just and the damned?"[11]

Many of these problems bear on the basic issue of objectivity versus subjectivity in historical writing. And unlike nineteenth-century "scientific historians," few today have any certainty they can write "objective history," even though they cannot abandon the goal.

If the historian does approximate his "serenity of perspective," he does it at a certain cost, for as George Kennan has pointed out, writing history represents "a certain turning one's back on the interests and preoccupations of one's own age, in favor of another . . . something which one's contemporaries, polite as they may be, rarely really understand or forgive. . . . The very idea that one of the members of this generation should turn away from its absorbing and unprecedented concerns to give his attention, professionally and at length, to the affairs of people who suffer from the obvious inferiority of not being alive at all . . . is little short of insulting."[12]

The Social Historian's Use of Psychology and Psychiatry

One of the most brilliant American historians of our generation, John Higham, noted that while the elderly Charles A. Beard, in the last few weeks of his life, "still insisted, 'Economics explains the mostest!'" he added, after a pause: "But I may have neglected the irrational."[13] Higham goes on to mention that World War II set many others thinking about irrational motivations in history.

During the 1920s, Freud's concepts of unconscious motivation began to attract American intellectuals. In 1925, the distinguished American historian, Harry Elmer Barnes, published a short book entitled *Psychology and History,* in which he pointed out: "Within the last few years there have been discoveries and advances in psychology which are of such far-reaching importance and so revolutionary a nature that they threaten the well-nigh total discrediting of the conventional historical literature, insofar as it touches individuals and their motives."[14] Historians, however, did not rush to adopt such insights or seriously attempt to cope with the irrational in history. As Higham has pointed out, the reluctance of historians to "accept the non-rational as a legitimate and persuasive dimension of reality" was linked to an acceptance of the doctrine of human progress. Such a belief has to assume "that men are rational: [that] they ordinarily pursue their individual or collective self-interest, and such self-interest is either rationally perceived or—at worst—coherently rationalized."[15]

From Freud onward, psychiatrists have had no reluctance to publish psychoanalytical biographical studies, but then they did not have to cope with the professional historian's rigor of documentation. One of the more entertaining biographical studies, by a psychiatrist and of a historian, is James Lorimer Halliday's *Mr. Carlyle My Patient: A Psychosomatic Biography*.[16] Halliday, who lived in Glasgow, became interested in Thomas Carlyle because of his life-long record of bodily complaints—abdominal pains, indigestion, migraine, etc., for which his physicians found no organic cause. Dr. Halliday, who fortunately writes with considerable humor, concludes his diagnosis with: "This is a compulsive 'anal' character of high intelligence and with definite paranoid traits of inflation and self-isolation, marked sadistic and masochistic tendencies, and schizoid features . . . who suffers from periodical phases of depression and passivity when he is disinclined to do anything. . . . He has a hypochondriacal preoccupation with his gastrointestinal tract—when his depressions left he becomes [sic] productive—almost hypomanic." Halliday strongly recommended further observation with a view to psychotherapy for his illustrious patient.

Not until the 1950s did political and social historians begin to see the possibility of using insights from dynamic psychiatry in considering irrational motivation in history.[17] And even though in his 1957 presidential address to the American Historical Association, William L. Langer, the eminent political and diplomatic historian, challenged his colleagues to incorporate psychoanalytic understanding in their history, few historians have followed his advice.[18] The handful who have drawn upon psychoanalytic insights, have at best been quite restrained in their interpretations, as, for example, Alexander and Juliette George in *Woodrow Wilson and Colonel House: A Personality Study*.[19] Perhaps the most penetrating biographic study based on psychoanalytic theory has been written not by a historian but by the psychoanalyst Erik H. Erikson: *The Young Man Luther: A Study in Psychoanalysis and History*.[20]

The historian faces numerous problems in trying to utilize psychodynamic concepts to interpret historical figures. He must first acquire a thorough knowledge of psychoanalytic literature. This can be done through broad reading, but his understanding will be greatly heightened if he has gone through some psychotherapy, personal psychoanalysis, or formal analytic training. The central problem concerns the availability of documentary evidence to substantiate his insights. How much evidence should be accumulated before he attempts to diagnose conscious or unconscious elements of a personality pattern? It is, for example, notably difficult to locate documentation on the childhood of persons who subsequently develop into pivotal personages of their time. And yet, the tenets of dynamic psychiatry stress the crucial importance of the earliest years in character formation.

While few historians have embraced psychodynamic interpretations, Freud and his successors have made them chary of accepting avowedly conscious motivation as the determinant of behavior in history.

More historians have made use of insights from social psychology to deal historically with matters such as social mobility, the role of the family in political and social developments, and status consciousness. Abraham S. Eisenstadt, in "American History and the Social Sciences,"[21] singled out eight social and economic studies in American history published from 1951 on that utilize concepts of social psychology and other social sciences, among them Oscar Handlin's *The Uprooted* (1951), and John Higham's *Strangers in the Land* (1955).[22]

An area of history that fascinates both social historians and psychiatric historians is national character. The concept of national character has pervaded a large portion of American historical writing since the Revolutionary era. Some of the core influences on the development of this concept were set forth in an essay by Arthur Schlesinger, Sr., "What then is the American, this new man?," originally published in 1943 and reissued after World War II.[23] Schlesinger saw the American character emerging from an interplay of Old World influences and New World conditions, and pointed out many characteristics accepted as "American": the strong habit of work, indifference to aesthetic conditions, mechanical ingenuity, resourcefulness, creative energy, a tradition of wasteful living bred by an environment of plenty, the high scarcity value of women, social mobility, ingrained belief in equality of opportunity, individualistic bias, optimism, ease at overstatement. Schlesinger also explores the modifications in national character brought on by urbanism in the last half of the nineteenth century.

It is, then, not surprising that following World War II, with the emergence of a new U.S. national identity in world affairs, historians began a new exploration of national character and national values. Research in social psychology and cultural anthropology added further dimensions to the historian's research. Of the many studies that followed the war,[24] one of the most provocative was David M. Potter's *People of Plenty*.[25] Potter drew heavily on research from the behavioral sciences in this historical analysis of American character, in which he traced the national character to economic abundance.

SOCIAL HISTORY AND THE HISTORY OF PSYCHIATRY

Relatively few psychiatrists today would view the history of their field as a technical specialty bearing little or no relationship to the society in which they live. The social historian has difficulty perceiving how the history of psychiatry, in any age, can be viewed without a knowledge of the historical forces that fashioned the period. The historical role of democratic influences and the theme of struggle between the under-privileged and over-privileged, for example, inevitably enter into historical analyses of hospitalization and community care for mental patients, of the type of treatment available to different economic groups, and of the psychiatric profession. Unquestionably, there are areas of psychiatric history that the psychiatrist, with long experience in clinical situations, is uniquely equipped to handle. The social history attempting any value judgment on the effectiveness of psychiatric treatment, for example, can only rely on contemporary medical perspective and the testimony of expert witnesses. Only a small number of social historians are equipped by training to write knowledgeably on biological components of mental illness.

Relatively few professional historians have ventured directly into the history of psychiatry, and their number has not increased substantially in recent years. The few book-length studies written by historians include Gerald Grob's *The State and the Mentally Ill* (1966) and *Mental Institutions in America* (1973), Norman Dain's *Concepts of Insanity in the United States, 1789–1865* (1964), and John Burnham's, *Psychoanalysis and American Medicine, 1894–1918* (1967).[26] Several articles on the subject have been written by such historians as Charles Rosenberg, Dorothy Ross, and Jeanne Brand.

Among the areas in psychiatric history to which the social historian may bring particular competence are the provision of hospitalization and community care; local, state, and national responsibility for services to the mentally ill; psychiatry as a professional field; legislation for the mentally ill; and the psychiatric parameters of social movements and social change.

The psychiatrist who draws upon the methodology of professional historians will approach the history of his field with sharpened perceptions. The historian who is able to utilize psychiatric concepts judiciously in viewing the past can write better history. Certainly each has much to gain in the sharing of their experience.

REFERENCES

1. Arthur S. Schlesinger, Jr., "The Historian and History," in *The Craft of American History: Selected Essays*, edited by Abraham S. Eisenstadt (New York: Harper & Row, 1966), Vol. I, p. 102.
2. Louis Gottschalk, Clyde Kluckhohn, and Robert Angell, eds., *The Use of Personal Documents in History, Anthropology, and Sociology*, Social Science Research Council Bulletin 53 (New York: Social Science Research Council, 1945) pp. 8–10.

3. Pieter Geyl, *The Use and Abuse of History* (New Haven: Yale University Press, 1955), p. 611.

4. Sir Charles Oman, *On the Writing of History* (New York: E. P. Dutton, 1939), pp. 206–211.

5. L. Gottschalk et al., op. cit. (in reference 2), p. 28ff. A useful text on the history of medicine is Edwin Clarke's *Modern Methods in the History of Medicine* (London: Athlone Press, 1971). For further general background on historical methodology, see also: Louis Gottschalk, *Understanding History: A Primer of Historical Method* (New York: Alfred A. Knopf, 1954); Marc Bloch, *The Historian's Craft* (New York: Alfred A. Knopf, 1953), passim. (This book was originally published in French in 1941 as *Apologie pour l'histoire, ou metier d'historien*); H. C. Hockett, *The Critical Method in Historical Research and Writing* (New York: Macmillan, 1955), pp. 13–72; Gaetano Salvemini, *History and Scientist: An Essay on the Nature of History and the Social Sciences* (Cambridge, Harvard University Press, 1939), passim; W. B. Wilcox, "An Historian Looks at Social Change," in Eisenstadt, op. cit. (in reference 1), pp. 24–32. A manual that has value for researchers in many disciplines is: Jacques Barzun and Henry F. Graff, *The Modern Researcher* (New York: Harcourt, Brace & World, 1957).

6. Bloch, op. cit. (in reference 5), pp. 97–112.

7. Robin G. Collingwood, *The Idea of History* (Oxford: Clarendon Press, 1946), p. 282. See also on this point Edward H. Carr, *What Is History?* (London: Macmillan, 1962), pp. 17–19.

8. Sidney Hook, for example, in *The Hero in History—A Study in Limitation and Possibility* (New York: John Day, 1943), p. 229, observes that "if the hero is defined as an event-making individual who redetermines the course of history, democratic societies must be eternally on guard against him. . . . For in such a society leadership cannot arrogate to itself heroic powers."

9. H. G. Wells as cited in Geoffrey Barraclough, *History in a Changing World* (New York: Oxford University Press, 1955), p. 225.

10. Herbert Butterfield, *History and Human Relations* (London: Collins, 1951), p. 114.

11. Bloch, op. cit. (in reference 5), p. 140.

12. George F. Kennan, "The Experience of Writing History" in Eisenstadt, op. cit. (in reference 1), Vol. II, p. 275.

13. John Higham et al., *History* (Englewood Cliffs, N.J.: Prentice Hall, 1965), p. 230.

14. Harry Elmer Barnes, *Psychology and History* (New York: Century, 1925), p. 73. Well before Barnes' interest, Karl Lamprecht (1856–1915), an economic historian from the University of Leipzig, in a series of lectures at Columbia University (1904) had urged historians to look to theoretical psychology in interpreting history. (Karl G. Lamprecht, *What Is History? Five Lectures on the Modern Science of History,* translated from the German by E. A. Andrews (New York:

Macmillan, 1905). First published in Germany in 1904 under the title *Moderne Geschichtswissenschaft.*

15. Higham et al., op cit. (in reference 13), p. 229. Professor Higham notes that two early studies by professional historians can be credited for introducing "a large, effective grasp of the non-rational elements in human conduct": Henry Nash Smith's *Virgin Land* (1950) and Richard Hofstadter's *American Political Tradition* (1948).

16. James Lorimer Halliday, *Mr. Carlyle My Patient: A Psychosomatic Biography,* (New York: Grune & Stratton, 1950), p. 81.

17. The Committee on Historiography of the Social Science Research Council, in preparing a report, *The Social Sciences in Historical Study* (New York: Social Science Research Council, 1954), examined the place of social psychology in history. The committee felt that psychological considerations entered into explanations of human action at two points in diagnosing the facts and in the selection of explanatory principles. Although regretting the "somewhat barbarous vocabulary" the historian had to familiarize himself with in order to understand psychology, the committee acknowledged that such considerations were particularly valuable in the psychology of leadership and in biographical studies. But they pointed to the great methodological difficulties involved, observing that: "Explanations of the behavior of an individual in terms of certain personal qualities imputed to him without independent evidence as to how he acquired or developed such qualities do not constitute sound practice, if only for the reason that they cannot be proved or disproved." (Ibid., p. 68.)

18. William L. Langer, "The Next Assignment," *American Historical Review,* 63 (Jan. 1952), pp. 284–288. For further discussion on this overall subject, see Fritz Schmidl, "Psychoanalysis and History," *Psychoanalytic Quarterly, 31* No. 4 (1962), pp. 532–548; Bruce Mazlish, ed., *Psychoanalysis and History* (Englewood Cliffs, N.J.: Prentice-Hall, 1963), and "Inside the Whales," *The Times Literary Supplement,* July 28, 1966, pp. 667-669; Raymond de Saussure, "Psychoanalysis and History," in *Psychoanalysis and the Social Sciences,* edited by Geza Roheim (New York: International Universities Press, 1947–51), Vol. 2, pp. 7–64; Franz Alexander, "Psychology and the Interpretation of Historical Events," in *The Cultural Approach to History,* edited by C. F. Ware (New York: Columbia University Press, 1940).

19. Alexander George and Juliette George, *Woodrow Wilson and Colonel House: A Personality Study* (New York: John Day, 1956). See also in this respect, Page Smith, *The Historian and History* (New York: Random House, 1966), pp. 124–128. Professor Smith cites two other biographies of superior quality that claim to utilize psychoanalytic insights: Emery Battis' study of Anne Hutchinson, *Saints and Sectaries* [sic] (Chapel Hill: University of North Carolina, 1962), and Fawn Brodie's *Thaddeus Stevens, Scourge of the South* (New York: W. W. Norton, 1959). See also John A. Garraty, *The Nature of Biography* (New York, Random House, 1957), and Garraty's article, "The Inter-

relations of Psychology and Biography," *Psychological Bulletin*, 51 (Nov. 1954), pp. 569–582. To these could also be added David Donald's *Charles Summer and the Coming of the Civil War* (New York: Knopf, 1960), and William Wilcox and Frederick Wyatt's, "Sir Henry Clinton: A Psychological Exploration in History," *William and Mary Quarterly* 3rd Series, 16 (1959), pp. 3–26.

20. Erik H. Erikson, *The Young Man Luther: A Study in Psychoanalysis and History* (New York: Norton, 1958).

21. Eisenstadt, op. cit. (in reference 1), pp. 24–32.

22. Ibid., p. 114.

23. Arthur M. Schlesinger, Sr., "What, then, is the American, this new man?," *American Historical Review*, 48 (1943), pp. 225–244. Republished in *Paths to the Present*, rev. ed. (Boston: Houghton Mifflin, 1964; 1st edition, 1949). John Higham attributes the revival of serious consideration of national character to Margaret Mead's *And Keep Your Powder Dry* (1942). (Higham et all., *History*, op. cit. (in reference 13) p. 221.)

24. See, for example, Oscar Handlin, *This Was America* (Cambridge: Harvard University Press, 1949); Henry S. Commager, *America in Perspective: The U.S. Through Foreign Eyes* (New York: Random House, 1947); Clyde Kluckhohn, "Have there been discernible shifts in American values during the past generation?" in *The American Style*, edited by E. E. Morison (Harper, 1958; Kluckhohn includes an excellent bibliography of recent literature); Louis Kronenberger, *Company Manners: A Cultural Inquiry into American Life* (Indianapolis: Bobbs Merrill, 1954); Max Lerner, *America as a Civilization* (New York: Simon and Schuster, 1957); Ralph Barton Perry, *Characteristically American* New York: Knopf, 1949); Warren S. Tyron, *A Mirror for Americans: Life and Manners in the United States, 1790–1870, as Recorded by American Travellers*, 3 vols. (Chicago: University of Chicago Press, 1952).

25. David M. Potter, *People of Plenty* (Chicago: University of Chicago Press, 1954).

26. Gerald Grob, *The State and the Mentally Ill: A History of Worcester State Hospital in Massachusetts, 1830–1920* (Chapel Hill: University of North Carolina Press, 1966), and *Mental Institutions in America: Social Policy to 1875* (New York: Free Press; London: Collier Macmillan, 1973); Norman Dain, *Concepts of Insanity in the United States, 1789–1865* (New Brunswick, N.J.: Rutgers University Press, 1964); and John Burnham, *Psychoanalysis and American Medicine, 1894–1918, Medicine, Science and Culture* (New York: International Universities Press, 1967, *Psychological Issues*, Vol. 5, No. 4).

Rudolph E. Siegel

2

Complementary Approach
to Medical Historiography

*At every moment of history man has to rewrite the history
of mankind.*

—Walther Riese
The Conception of Disease: Its History,
Its Versions and Its Nature

Most modern physicists are convinced that the phenomena they observe are events of an outside world independent of our existence and that the recognition of these events is subject to modification by the process of observation. Similarly, the approach of historians is affected by personal preferences, involving the selection and the form of presentation of historical material. Buchdahl[1] wrote in a review of two publications concerning a revolution in the historiography of science: "It is not possible to isolate opinions concerning scientific knowledge from questions of the validity of the ideas that are involved in the general concept of knowledge." Walther Riese, a medical historian of deep philosophical interests, pointed out that "even those who cherish the idea or illusion of an impersonal and anonymous science do not escape the law of a personal equation, be it only for the selection of the material offered."[2]

In addition, because of an increasing trend among medical historians to discourage the search for similarities or analogies between ancient and contemporary thought, the tracing of modern medical concepts back to ideas and doctrines of a time more distant than a few decades has lately been frowned upon. To support the exclusion of this method, historians have pointed to the unique character of each cultural climate; such a detached representation of historical events, however, would fail to illuminate many sources of present-day

14

thought and would prevent historians from demonstrating the continuity and evolution of science. The newly suggested term "presentism" discourages much historical inquiry by discrediting the search for similarities of thought during successive periods; it also denounces the current tendency "of exclusively evaluating older doctrines in terms of present knowledge."

The current doctrine favoring environmental and purely cultural factors is thus liable to draw the attention of the reader away from the study of the basic concepts of earlier times. On the other hand, a more comprehensive approach suggests that the historical motives of earlier opinions and discoveries should not be "narrowly conceived from a twentieth-century point of view . . . nor seen foreshortened from the retrospective viewpoint of the twentieth century."[3] We should, therefore, search for the roots and influences that determine particular events of the past, and should elaborate on the undeniable influence of personalities or issues on later generations. Without an awareness of such frequently far-reaching influences it would be difficult to teach any continuity in the history of ideas.

The branches of science that have contributed most to medical advances are represented by natural science in general, botany as the foundation of ancient drug therapy, mathematics, and philosophy, as well as logic; these are only a few of the disciplines once mandatory for the young physician. Agassi, in a study of the philosophy of history,[4] stated: "The broad outline of the history of science is the history of the choice of central problems and of the various schools of thought which attempted to answer these problems." Agassi stressed that earlier scientists had overlooked certain facts and ideas not only because of technical difficulties but because of the shortcomings of their scientific theories. The historian should point out such past errors and recognize the difficulties faced by our predecessors.

We are reminded of the continuity of tradition by the fact that most modern medical concepts are expressed in Greek and Latin. Furthermore, modern physicians and medical scientists react much like their predecessors to the same situations and questions, since they face more or less the same observations and problems. The fundamental processes of human thought have not really changed. Moreover, medical history should not be written as a smooth account of discoveries, since most inventions and opinions contain errors and inconsistencies that should be pointed out. Many great discoveries owe their origin to a person's attempt to clear up apparent contradictions, for instance, the changing interpretation of the concepts of matter, air (pneuma), irritability, reflex and instinct, the nature of the soul, and biological forces.

The approach of earlier scientists often has a metaphysical taint, as is evident in the question of the stability of species. The ancients, especially Aristotle and Galen, insisted that all organisms grow according to a fixed design developed by a higher mind, often called *demiourgos* (craftsman), who was thought to have fashioned an integrated plan for all living species as well as for their environment. Since adaptation was predestined, the "unfit" fell by the wayside; selection was not the decisive factor for the survival of better-adapted species.[5] We thus have to reconstruct the metaphysical and often the religious background of earlier scientists in order to understand their motivation, for such considerations can either support or retard scientific advance.

Although the variety of medical doctrines arose from different approaches to the formulation of problems and their solution, an almost unbroken chain of medical thought and physiological doctrines can be found by studying the changing concept of disease. We always have to keep in mind that most symptoms presented to physicians by their patients have remained unchanged through time, in contrast to shifting methods of interpretation. Thus, it might be well to encourage a twofold, complementary method of writing medical history in the manner of optical perspective, like the painter who connects the foreground by lines to the vanishing point. That is, we should approach a historical problem in a dual fashion, by looking forward and backward. These views are complementary and mutually supporting.

Humanistic studies contain little support for those who condemn the far-reaching backward look of the historian. For instance, linguists examine subtle changes in the meaning of terms and phrases over the course of centuries. In many cases the original meaning of these expressions has been modified or enriched but not abolished by the superimposition of new associations. Riese has correctly stated this tradition: "The number of nervous diseases the names of which reflect a functional approach is very small, and they belong to the ancient treasure of neurology."[6]

Retrospection is also evident in the terminology of philosophers and psychologists who have recognized the influence of ancient doctrines on today's ideas. Rather than smugly stating that such an interpretation implies "projecting modern scientific concepts and problems onto writers of classical antiquity," we should admit seeing the ancient authors as precursors of contemporary scientific development[7]; one of the most attractive aspects of historiography is the demonstration of the evolution of ideas.

No less an authority than Ludwig Edelstein wrote in a review of Cohen and Drabkin's *A Sourcebook in Greek Science*:[8] "In mathematics, astronomy, and mathematical geography, the Greek developed and followed methods that closely approximate . . . the standards of modern science. . . . The link between the ancient investigations and those of modern times is obvious."[9] He also pointed out that many ancient authors were guided in their research by philosophical theories: "In fact, evaluating the tension between the various tendencies within ancient science is one of the main problems confronting the historian."[10] Edelstein's advice that "the achievements of the ancients have to be seen in their own setting"[11] does not at all contradict his statement that "one type of Greek scientific argument is strikingly similar to modern science,"[12] for modern science and ancient science are not diametrically opposed.

A continuous development is most evident in the history of the physical sciences and astronomy. Observations became more exact with the advance of technology; new mathematical concepts rendered physical laws more accurate and applicable to a larger field of observations. Consequently, older laws became invalid, remaining useful only as crude approximations, although they had been useful previously in a different historical setting. Thus, while Aristarchus of Samos (280 B.C.) postulated a heliocentric solar system, he was unable to prove his intuition either because of insufficient evidence, methodological difficulties, or the prejudice of his contemporaries. Since the essence of "discovery consists not in formulation of a concept but rests on convincing proof," he cannot be credited with the "discovery" of the heliocentric doctrine of astronomy. Similarly, nobody would accuse a historian of impermissible hindsight for describing the circular orbits of the Copernican system as an approximation to the true elliptical orbits demonstrated by Kepler.

The principle of an unbroken advance applies equally to the history of the biological sciences. Hippocrates expressed this idea in his treatise *On Ancient Medicine* when he wrote: "Full discovery will be made if the inquirer is competent and conducts his researches with knowledge of the discoveries already made."[13]

In the quest to explain the circulation of blood, the first step was taken at the time of Hippocrates with the discovery of the one-way mechanism of the cardiac valves. Then Galen proved that blood was contained in both arteries and veins, and that it was fallacious to believe in the presence of air in the arteries. Harvey took the third, decisive step by establishing that venous blood flows toward the heart but not in the opposite direction. He thus eliminated the last fundamental error in the basic concepts of blood flow. With the microscopical demonstration of capillaries by Malpighi, the final principle of the circulatory system was established.

Following ancient preconceptions, Harvey related circulation to distillation, since he put heat production in the heart, the "hearth" of the body, comparable to the sun of the universe. In *De motu cordis*, Harvey repeatedly mentioned Galen's reference to a pulmonary transit of blood, and incorporated many positive aspects of earlier doctrines in his final argument for a circular blood flow. Only a detailed retrospective view can make us fully appreciate the genius of earlier physiologists and their shortcomings—such as, for instance, the inexplicable oversight by the ancients of the role speed and pressure play in the flow of blood, despite the competent work in hydraulics done by Hero of Alexandria.

Another example of the two-way complementary approach to medical historiography is represented by the fundamental distinction between successive doctrines of nerve conduction. Earlier periods favored a preponderantly deductive approach, in contrast to the later prevalence of the inductive and experimental approach.

Galen thought that a nervous stimulus was transmitted either by a pneuma originally present in the nerve or entering the nerve from the brain at the exact moment of stimulation. He left it undecided whether the penuma propagating such a stimulus was of a material or immaterial nature. He further suggested that the strength of such a stimulus either maintains its full intensity during passage from the brain through the spinal cord to the active muscle, or triggers a proportionally much stronger reaction (*auxetrenai*, amplified), manifested by a powerful contraction of the muscle.

Since Galen believed in the importance of material qualities, he supplemented the earlier purely mechanistic pneumatic doctrine with prechemical concepts. For the first time, he differentiated the stimulation of nerves from the associated changes that take place in the muscle during contraction by relating the cause of the active change (*drastike kinesis;* literally, active motion) to the contractile faculty (*dynamis*) of the muscle, but he connected the propagation of stimuli to the conductive faculty of the nerve. Galen's description of the conductive power of the nerve anticipated the modern concept of stimulus,[14] although the Greeks had no specific term for stimulus.

Galen had followed Aristotle by defining every change in an organ as movement (*kinesis*). Since neither Aristotle nor Galen supported an atomistic concept of matter, they applied the term kinesis not only to spatial displacement but also to qualitative changes. In modern biology, a spatial movement of chemical compounds through cells or across membranes that leads to structural, electrical, or chemical changes results in qualitative alteration (*alloiosis*) of the substrate. Thus, this ancient doctrine of stimulation and nerve conduction

was an early attempt to establish a relationship between spatial movement and qualitative alteration of tissues.

Later authors attempted to construct mechanical models of this
biological mechanism. In the eighteenth century, the discovery of
chemical compounds suggested a propagation of chemical reactions
through a hollow nerve; this doctrine replaced the earlier mechanical
idea of an advancing wave of pneuma or nerve spirit (also called
Nervenkraft).

When electricity became known as a potentially stimulating force
for biological systems, its physiological role was initially denied. Johannes Mueller (1801–1858) spoke of the poorly defined principle of
Nervenkraft. Apparently the influence of the Galenic doctrine of
pneuma had not yet waned, although Mueller did not compare Nervenkraft with pneuma.[15]

Similarly, the definition of diseases has been subject to a con-
tinuously changing evaluation of etiology and the importance of certain clinical symptoms, a fact that is borne out by a review of the
changing interpretation of heart diseases, the true nature of which
long remained unrecognized.

Galen accounted for affections of the heart in the chapter on
respiratory ailments in his great clinical work, De locis affectis.[16] His
attention was completely focused on the combustive (respiratory)
process that allegedly produced the vital animal heat in the left cardiac ventricle. Galen observed that patients often succumbed shortly
after cardiac injuries received in combat when the blood was drained
from the arterial system. Otherwise, "an affection of the heart did not
appear as cause of shortness of breath besides the types mentioned
in the treatise On dyspnoea."[17] However, "When the heart is over-
heated it renders respiration deep and frequent. . . . If, contrary to
this, the heart suffers from cooling, respiration becomes shallow and
slow."[18] Galen related sudden death to undercooling of the heart or
to other humoral causes but not to structural changes.

Galen was also aware that unidentified changes in the heart occasionally caused clinical symptoms: "Sudden attacks of palpitation
of the heart can be seen in many young people who are in perfect
health and in others past their prime without any other evident
symptoms. . . . Some do collapse . . . after a certain period of good
health. . . . The majority of the persons thus affected were of an age
of less than fifty but more than forty years."[19]

Galen followed the traditional concept of sympathy in attributing the associated severe pain in the lower chest to secondary (sympathetic) involvement of the lower esophagus or of the upper end of
the stomach (cardia). He could not visualize a primary involvement

of the heart muscle itself, because of the old superstition that the heart was the seat of the soul. Even later physicians, while rejecting this doctrine, failed to recognize intrinsic diseases of the heart. Since the term *cardia* indicated both the heart and the esophagealgastric junction, the differential diagnostic discussion remained confusing.[20] Medieval and Renaissance physicians occasionally found calcifications of the coronary arteries on autopsy of people who had died from dropsy or had suffered instant death. In 1776, Heberden convincingly described *angina pectoris,*[21] but Heberden still failed to associate this condition and its lethal consequences with coronary calcification. Not until 1912 did Herrick describe the classical triad of angina pectoris, coronary sclerosis, and myocardial infarction in his paper "Clinical Features of Sudden Obstruction of the Coronary Arteries."[22]

The complete reversal of the explanation of this clinical syndrome deserves examination; Galen thought that sudden death, especially of middle-aged men under fifty, suffering from acute chest pain and syncope, resulted from respiratory standstill. He attributed the cessation of heartbeat and pulse to a sudden extinction of combustion in the left ventricle due to a severe humoral disturbance or sympathetic irritation of the organ in this area of the body. Today we know that the cessation of respiration results from a sudden stoppage of the heartbeat. Correspondingly, we attribute death by *asphyxia* to the lack of air, secondary to heart disease, whereas the ancients understood asphyxia as pulselessness (*sphygmos,* pulse), secondary to a standstill of intracardiac ventilation and combustion.

These accounts should suffice to demonstrate that our interpretation of older descriptions of this syndrome is certainly not a "pretty, stained artifact," as one critic called the interpretation of earlier medical history in the light of modern clinical knowledge. Yet other questions have been raised about the value of retrospective interpretation. Walter Pagel warned that those who reconstruct the thought of a historical personality in its original setting will encounter two sets of thought, a scientific and a nonscientific type.[23] These should be "conceived in spite of each other and as an inorganic whole in which they support and confirm each other,"[24] even though some of the older facts may appear to the historian as "useless and unscientific."[25] This statement certainly points in the right direction. But should we, with Pagel, really declare certain ideas of older scientists "useless and unscientific," regardless of whether or not ancient authors were aware of questionable aspects in their doctrines? Rather than assessing the value of earlier scientists' opinions, should we not consider their shortcomings and contradictions as the starting point for subsequent constructive work?

Such a situation, for instance, can be found in the history of the doctrine of vision.[26] Since Galen did not see how rectilinear light rays could follow the curved path of the optic nerve from eye to brain, he explained this section of the visual pathway by a purely pneumatic transmission, but still held to a geometrical explanation of squint and diplopia that seemed to require a straight projection of the image from object to brain.

In a similar manner, Galen accounted for discrepancies in the doctrines of respiration and blood flow by postulating a reflux of toxic fumes against the stream of aerated blood through the mitral valve into the pulmonary vein and lungs. In this instance, the mechanistic aspect of flow was subordinated to a faulty respiratory doctrine postulating a leakage from the mitral valve. He accepted these inconsistencies in order to maintain a uniform theory of respiration.

Further epistemological errors are manifest in the invention of additional assumptions to explain discrepancies in doctrines that could not account for all observations but were still maintained. In earlier times, such controversies remained sterile until new experimental techniques were invented. Modern investigators are more aware that apparently divergent results in their own experimental work often point to an incorrect, preconceived doctrine; this opens an avenue to additional research.

To consider ultimately disproved postulates of science as useless and unworthy of mentioning constitutes a retrospective judgment that a historian cannot afford, for the goals and definitions of research have changed repeatedly. Lindholm[27] suggested that we be aware of metaphysical theories influencing the formulation of past doctrines and try to understand the hidden assumptions of historical concepts. Still, we cannot expect that earlier science will present a coherent system of thought.

In a paper on the classification of neurological diseases, Riese[28] stressed the difficulty of this task, since he was aware that "the common feature of the classification of nervous diseases is the total lack of a uniform principle of classification." He pointed out that the history of nervous diseases cannot be presented objectively and impartially since an impersonal and anonymous science does not exist. He was conscious of the intrusion of a personal equation in the selection of the material offered, and realized that our own standard of values cannot be completely separated from our presentation of historical facts.

No one from the twentieth century is able to consider older medical inventions, doctrines, or clinical diagnoses exclusively from the values and viewpoints of past times. In addition, younger physicians will become interested in the history of our profession only if we connect the advances leading to present-day knowledge with the endeavors and thoughts of earlier periods. We, therefore, must approach historiography with prospection and retrospection, in consideration of both the ancient sources and the ever-advancing goal of the healing arts. Present-day science is only a transitional phase in a continuous evolution. By employing a complementary working method, we can keep medical history from being cut off from the living tree of modern medicine and science of which it represents a vital branch.

In recognition of this concept, O. Temkin wrote: "If medical ideas are merely treated as phenomena or products of their time, their medical truth too might appear to be restricted to their respective periods. . . . The danger lies in the assumption that cultures, periods or social classes are closed, self-centered entities, an assumption which, in the final analysis, would make historical studies senseless. . . ."[29]

As Riese stated:

> A concept cannot be made the subject of a tale; it has to be analyzed. Though disease is a basic experience of human existence, each stage of civilization has its own concept of disease. But it would not be possible to write the history of the various concepts of disease as the unbroken line of a chapter of human thought leading in the irreversible march of time from the most primitive and crudest magic thought to the most refined and elaborate concept of modern psychology. In fact, the various concepts of disease have always been overlapping, living side by side at each stage of human history, and the road from primitive to rational thought has to be sought and rediscovered anew by each generation and each individual. Nor is any generation or any individual protected against the danger of relapsing into early concepts, once the final stage is reached. At every moment of his history man has to rewrite the history of mankind. Thus emerges the plan of the history of omni-present ideas rather than that of events and discoveries happening but once.[30]

REFERENCES

1. G. Buchdahl, "A revolution in historiography of science" (book review), *Hist. Sci.*, 4:55, 1974.
2. W. Riese, *A history of neurology*, M.D. Monographs of medical history (New York: M.D. Publications, 1959).
3. K. D. Keele (book review), *Med Hist.*, 18:305, 1974.
4. J. Agassi, "History and theory: Studies in the philosophy of history," in *Towards an historiography of science* (S'Gravenhage, The Netherlands: Mouton & Co., 1963), Suppl. 2, pp. 27, 53.

5. M. J. Kottler, "Alfred Russell Wallace, the origin of man, and spiritualism," *Isis*, 65:145–192, 1974.
6. W. Riese, "History and principles of classification of nervous diseases," *Bull. Hist. Med.*, 18:465–512, 1945, 496.
7. L. G. Ballester (book review), *Clio Med.*, 9:264–266 1974.
8. L. R. Cohen and I. L. Drabkin, *A source book in Greek science* (Cambridge: Harvard Univ. Press, 1958).
9. L. Edelstein, "Recent trends in the interpretation of ancient science," P. P. Wiener and A. Noland, *Roots of scientific thought* (New York: Basic Books, 1958), p. 91.
10. L. Edelstein, op. cit. (in reference 9), p. 95, 96.
11. Ibid., p. 113.
12. Ibid., p. 119.
13. Hippocrates, Greek text with English translation by W. H. S. Jones (London: Heinemann, 1923), vol. 1, p. 15.
14. R. E. Siegel, *Galen on psychology, psychopathology, and function and diseases of the nervous system* (Basel: Karger, 1973), pp. 86, 88–90.
15. K. E. Rothschuh, *Vom spiritus animalis zum Nervenaktionstrom;* Ciba Zeitschrift #89, Band 8 (Basel: Ciba, 1958), pp. 2950–2955.
16. Galen, "De locis affectis," in Galen, *Opera omnia*, ed. by D. C. G., Kuehn, (Leipzig: Cnobloch, 1821–1833), vol. 8, pp. 1–452.
17. Galen, "De difficultate respirationis," in *Opera omnia*, op. cit. (in reference 16), vol. 7, pp. 753–960.
18. Galen, "De locis affectis" op. cit. (in reference 16), vol. 8, p. 306.
19. Ibid., p. 305.
20. R. E. Siegel, *Galen's system of physiology and medicine: An analysis of his doctrines and observations on blood flow, respiration, humors and internal diseases* (Basel: Karger 1968), pp. 30, 344ff.
21. W. Heberden, *Commentaries on the history and cure of diseases* (London: Payne, 1802; reprint, New York: Hafner, 1962).
22. J. B. A. Herrick, "Clinical features of sudden obstruction of the coronary arteries," *J. Am. Med. Assoc.*, 59:2015–2020, 1912.
23. A. G. Debus, ed., *Science, medicine and society in the renaissance* (1972), Vol. 1, p. 7.
24. Ibid., p. 6.
25. R. E. Siegel, *Galen on sense perception* (Basel: Karger. 1970) p. 71ff, p. 106ff.
26. Ibid.
27. L. M. Lindholm in *Proceedings of the XXIII International Congress of the History of Medicine, London 1972* (London: Wellcome Institute Hist. Med., 1974), pp. 1099–1105.
28. W. Riese, op. cit. (in reference 6).
29. O. Temkin, "The historiography of ideas in medicine," in E. Clarke, ed., *Modern methods in the history of science* (London: Athlone Press, 1971), p. 12.
30. W. Riese, *The conception of disease, its history, its versions and its nature,* (New York: Philosophical Library, 1953), forward.

Ernst Fischer

3

Vacillating Conceptions on the Use of Electrical Stimulation in Muscle Paralysis*

On July 1, 1773, the well-known British scientist John Walsh wrote to Benjamin Franklin (who had described the electric nature of lightning in 1752), that he had established the electric nature of the shocks delivered by certain torpedo fishes. Torpedoes, and to a much lesser extent other species of electric fishes, were known to the ancient scholars, who even advocated their use for medical purposes. This bit of history has to be recalled here, since in accordance with Wilson's view (1857), one can regard the electric fishes as "the earliest electric mashines [sic] used by mankind."

The development of any realistic conception of why electrical stimulation might be beneficial in the treatment of muscular paralysis following nerve injuries depended on the historical development of our physiological knowledge as well as on our progressively improved technical equipment to produce different electric wave forms.

Albrecht von Haller discovered in 1743 not only that muscles could be activated by stimulation of their nerves, but that muscle fibers themselves have "irritability," since mechanical as well as chemical stimuli applied directly to them causes contraction. The relation between the strength of the stimulus and the strength of the resulting contraction remained rather mystical for a considerable period due to various, more or less secondary, factors that complicated the problem. Ritter, early in the nineteenth century, demonstrated clearly that

---

*Literature references can be obtained from E. Fischer, M.D., 3110 Manor Drive, Richmond, Va., 23230.

24

electrical stimuli directly applied to a skeletal muscle belong to five classes according to stimulus strength and the strength of the provoked contractions. He found, expressed in modern phraseology: (1) subthreshold or subliminal stimuli, too weak to produce any contraction; (2) a threshold or liminal stimulus as the weakest stimulus that can produce the smallest visible contraction; (3) submaximal stimuli, which are above threshold and which with increased strength cause increased contractions; (4) a well-defined maximal stimulus, which when further increased does not produce a stronger contraction; and (5) supramaximal stimuli, which are stronger than the maximal stimulus, but waste unnecessary electric energy.

Alexander von Humboldt was probably the first to employ the expressions "galvanism" and "galvanization" for the use of direct currents for stimulating purposes; these terms are still used in the physical therapy literature. However, the use of these terms should be avoided today since stimulating currents should be characterized according to shape, strength, and duration. Salandiere is reported to have been the first routinely to use direct currents for therapeutic purposes, stimulating human muscles by needles inserted through the skin.

Although direct currents were generally used to stimulate nerves and muscles in the eigtheenth century, the improvement of the static friction machine by the Scottish monk Gorden in 1742 and the somewhat later invention of the Leyden jar made it possible in the second half of the eighteenth century to use with ease static electricity for stimulating purposes. I. J. Krueger predicted in 1744 that electricity would be the best therapeutic procedure for paralyzed limbs. In the same year, Kratzenstein demonstrated and discussed the use of electricity with his medical students. Soon after the discovery of induced currents by Faraday in 1833, induction coils were used for stimulation of nerves and muscles. In the American literature, these instruments were often called "Harvard coils" by physiologists, and "wallplates" by clinicians and physical therapists; and the use of this type of current was often called "Faradism" or "Faradization." As soon as alternating currents became generally available after 1883, and high-frequency currents after 1886, they also were used in physiology and physical therapy. It was soon apparent that for all these different electric wave forms, exactly the same relation held true between the strength of the stimulus and the strength of the contractions evoked, as was described by Ritter for direct currents.

The medical literature from the middle of the nineteenth century until about 1910 contains numerous papers, some advocating the use of electricity as beneficial in treatment of muscular paralysis, some skeptical, but all these papers were based only on clinical impressions gained as a rule from a very limited number of patients and without any reported measurements and control observations.

Reid in 1841 was probably the first to investigate experimentally the effect of electrical stimulation on denervation atrophy in animals. In a few frogs, he sectioned the cauda equina on both sides, and stimulated the gastrocnemius muscle on one side with apparently weak direct currents for several weeks. He reported that the treated muscle was finally about twice the size of the untreated one. Reid's paper was cited for nearly 100 years as proof of the beneficial effect of electrical stimulation of paralyzed muscles. Unfortunately, we know now that denervation atrophy progresses rather slowly in the frog, and in all probability, the increased weight of the treated gastrocnemius was due to a training effect of the stimulation on a more or less still normal muscle. Such an effect can be produced on normal muscles by considerably weaker stimulation than is required for retardation of denervation atrophy by appropriate treatment.

Twelve years after Reid's famous paper was published, Brown-Sequard not only confirmed that electrical treatment prevents denervation atrophy in frog muscles, but claimed that he was able to prevent atrophy in muscles of dogs, guinea pigs, rabbits, and pigeons. He claimed that even when atrophy was well developed, galvanism could gradually diminish the difference between the denervated muscle and the normal muscle on the other side, until the treated denervated muscle was as large as the normal muscle. As will be discussed later, no one in modern times has been able by any treatment to prevent denervation atrophy completely; all one is able to do is to retard its progress considerably. Apparently, Brown-Sequard did not prevent regeneration of the cut nerves, which, as is well known now, can reach the denervated muscle, reinnervate it, and lead to complete recovery. However, with such apparently excellent results, Brown-Sequard furthered considerably the use of galvanism in clinical practice. He himself claimed that in a patient with very far advanced lead palsy, the affected limb after electrical treatment became as strong as a normal limb. Obviously, today, we are more inclined to explain such a recovery by the prevention of further lead intake and by recovery or regeneration of the damaged motor nerves.

Since Reid and Brown-Sequard were recognized as the foremost medical scientists and clinicians of their time it is not astonishing that other physicians felt justified to claim, based on their own isolated impressions, the triumph of electrical treatment of muscular palsy. This affirmative period lasted nearly to the end of the nineteenth century, when Friedlander tried in 1896, somewhat in vain, to silence the slowly growing opposition to electrical treatment with a single experiment on one dog. He claimed that the weight of the treated muscle was higher than the corresponding muscle on the untreated side when both sciatic nerves were cut. There were a few other reports during that period, each on a limited number of animals; some had positive results, others were negative. They cannot be evaluated today, since the strength and the type of currents used, as well as the frequency and duration of the treatment sessions, were not reported adequately.

In 1913, the famous English physiologist Langley and his coworkers started to investigate the problem on a relatively large number of rabbits. Stimulating daily with condenser discharges, they found that the treated denervated muscles were only 10% heavier than the denervated control muscles. Their main conclusion was that denervation atrophy was caused by overwork due to denervation fibrillation of the muscle fibers. They concluded, furthermore, that fibrillation is responsible for the excess oxygen consumption of the denervated muscles, and that fibrillation was very little diminished by their treatment. Hartment and Blatz reported later that, even using somewhat stronger stimulation, the treatment minimally improved the power of the treated denervated muscles. For thirty years, therefore, denervation atrophy was regarded as an excess demand on the denervated muscle fibers and as primarily responsible for the quickly progressing atrophy. In 1940, Solandt and Maladery suppressed denervation fibrillation with quinine sulfate, and found that in the absence of fibrillation the rate of denervation atrophy was practically unaltered; they concluded that the atrophy was not caused by fibrillation.

Some neurologists of the nineteenth century realized that the excitability of the muscle alters progressively after denervation, but a true evaluation of changed muscle excitability became available only after it was understood that for an electrical stimulus to be effective and evoke contractions, not only its strength but also its duration was very important. Weiss in 1901 was one of the first to study the influence of strength and duration of rectangular currents for threshold stimulation. He constructed so-called strength-duration curves for various tissues. Very similar strength-capacity curves were obtained a few years later for condenser discharges with different voltage strengths and capacities, since the capacity determines the duration of the discharge. These and other experiments with different-shaped currents revealed that there is no single threshold stimulus; rather, each stimulus strength has its minimal duration, and each duration needs a minimal strength to cause threshold stimulation. The strength-duration curves for motor nerves and for muscle fibers revealed that for stimuli of short durations the nerve needs less current strength than does the muscle, while for stimuli of long durations the nerve needs a higher strength than does the muscle. Lapique, a pupil of Weiss, working on this problem since 1905, devised a practical solution in 1921 to compare the true excitability of various tissues. He recognized that for all the different tissues tested the shape of the strength-duration curves was identical, but their position in the co-ordinate system of voltage against time were distinctly different. It is typical for all strength-duration curves that beyond a certain duration of the stimulus, any further increase of duration requires the same voltage. In other words, for a duration longer than the "utilization time," the needed voltage remains constant, and some of the electrical current is wasted. This constant strength of stimuli of very long durations was called by Lapique the "rheobase." He demonstrated that the positions of all the strength-duration curves for various tissues could be characterized by what he called the "chronaxie." He defined chronaxie as the minimal time a stimulus of twice the rheobasic strength must last to be of threshold value. This doubling was not an arbitrary device, but was chosen because, of all possible threshold stimuli, one at roughly twice the rheobasic strength represented the threshold stimulus that required the minimal amount of electric energy. All threshold stimuli of longer or shorter durations than the chronaxie wasted a considerable amount of energy. Bourginion applied this principle extensively to normal and pathological human muscles, and demonstrated: (1) that the chronaxie has distinctly different ranges for the various anatomical muscles, and (2) that after denervation, chronaxie immediately lengthens to about twice the normal values, and furthermore lengthens rather progressively with the time elapsed since denervation.

These findings, which are of greatest importance for effective electrical treatment of denervated muscles, were neglected by clinicians for many years. It became apparent from these findings that by not using stimuli of chronaxie duration for electrical stimulation, one can apply to the muscle several times the energy necessary for maximal stimulation. That the application of too high an amount of electrical energy has a deteriorating effect on biological tissues, causing electrical burns, is well known even to the layman. For more than 100 years, the deteriorating effect of electricity was well known to physiologists, who warned students in their laboratories to avoid unnecessarily strong stimulation in their experimental work, since it could quickly kill the tissues they were trying to stimulate. Overstimulation has been used purposely by physiologists to kill quickly isolated muscles after myothermic measurements have been made. Nonreacting muscles were warmed with strong electrical shocks of known energy values, which enabled physiologists to calibrate immediately their experimental set-up.

The physiatrist Walthard emphasized in 1935 that any effective electrotherapy for muscular paralysis requires maximal muscle stimulation with rectangular currents of chronaxie duration and that single stimuli should be repeated at a frequency high enough to produce maximal tetanic contraction. He pleaded not too successfully that other physicians follow his advice. Henssge and Stark reported good results using direct currents of adjusted durations by utilizing, after necessary amplification, the action currents of quicker and slower muscles and even of smooth muscles, selected according to the chronaxie of the denervated muscles to be treated. The importance of maximal stimulation with minimal energies was often reiterated in later years and a number of clinical successes have been reported.

Clinical experience showed again and again that the use of optimal electrotherapy of denervated muscles was often extremely painful, especially when the nerve injury had affected the sensation of the limb only very little or not at all. Patients often refused to submit to further treatment. Therefore, it was proposed to compromise between minimal energy stimulation and less painful stimulation, by using some excess energy when stimulating the denervated muscles. Clinically sinusoidal currents of adequate frequencies, exponentially rising currents, and other current forms seemed better suited to this purpose than did the rectangular currents, which rise immediately to full strength.

When stimulating normal muscle to avoid disuse atrophy in a limb immobilized for a long time, the danger of painful stimulation is far less, since disused muscles retain the excitability of normal muscles and therefore need stimuli of only short duration to activate them. Debedat and Bordier were probably the first to use electrical stimulation routinely to prevent disuse atrophy.

Since graded electrical stimulation in animals can regulate the quantity of muscular activity, it has been used since 1927 with rabbits to correlate the changes in muscular metabolism with the amount of muscular activity. Besides the distinct weight increases of the treated normal muscles, the observed metabolic alterations were interpreted as an increase in the efficiency of the working metabolism and an increase in endurance. However, despite the increased diameter of the individual muscle fibers and the increased tension produced by the muscle, the tension per cross section of the muscle fibers and the birefringence of the fibers were not altered. When producing hypertrophy of normal muscle by electrical stimulation in cats, the hypertrophy was more pronounced for the flexor muscles than for the extensor muscles. The hypertrophy for both muscle groups was greater when during stimulation, the muscles were kept at a long-muscle length instead of at a short length.

Clinical observations have also shown that differences exist between the rate of atrophy for different muscles of the same person, and that the general rate of denervation atrophy is determined to a certain extent by hereditary conditions. Tower, in her classic paper of 1935 as well as in her review of 1939, showed that for the same species different muscles have different rates of denervation atrophy and that even for related mammalian species these rates may vary considerably. Her first statement was confirmed by other investigators in the case of cats and rabbits. However, for rats, the difference in denervation atrophy rates for various muscles was regarded as not statistically significant. Knowlton and Hines revealed in a careful study that the rate of denervation atrophy of the muscles of various mammalian species is correlated to the natural life-span of the species in question—the shorter the life-span, the more rapid the weight loss of denervation atrophy.

The interest of physiologists in electrical treatment of denervation atrophy was revived during World War II. It was then generally recognized that one had to study a large number of animals, if possible of uniform genetic origin, and that the experimental results had to be tested for statistical significance; to be effective, one had to use electrical stimuli adjusted to the excitability of the muscle to be treated. The first of this type of investigation was published by Fischer in 1939. Rats were denervated on both sides, but only one gastrocnemius was treated. The muscle was kept at a long-muscle length working against heavy resistance, while being electrically stimulated daily for 12 to 20 minutes with appropriate maximal currents. The muscle was stimulated for 1 minute with repeated shocks, producing maximal tetanic contractions several times in that period; this was followed by rest periods of 1 to 2 minutes, after which the stimulation-rest cycle was repeated. In order to use really maximal stimulation, it was necessary to keep the animals under light ether anesthesia during the stimulation session. Rats kept denervated for more than 4 weeks were reoperated after 23 to 26 days to prevent reinnervation of the muscles. The results demonstrated that this type of rigorous treatment retarded the lengthening of the chronaxie (the loss of excitability) distinctly, and retarded the loss in wet and dry weight of the muscles considerably; it also raised the increased oxygen consumption of the denervated muscles to a still higher level. In another series of tests, the muscles of both legs were electrically treated, but not with stimuli adjusted to their chronaxies. The muscles of one leg were stimulated with faradic currents of rather short duration, and the muscles of the other leg received rectangular currents of long duration. As expected, faradic stimulation was more effective for the first 2 weeks of denervation, and galvanic stimulation was more effective in subsequent weeks. Although appropriate electrical stimulation retarded denervation atrophy considerably, the gain in power corresponded roughly to the increased muscle weight. There was no increase in power calculated per cross-section unit of the muscle fibers. Birefringence measurements revealed that during denervation atrophy the alterations in submicroscopical structure had about the same time course as the loss in power per cross-section unit. Optical electrical treatment of denervated muscle was shown to have no influence on the deterioration of the submicroscopical structure. However, appropriate electrical treatment prevented potassium loss, which occurred otherwise after denervation, and it occasionally increased the potassium content of the treated muscle slightly above normal values. The sodium content, therefore, did not increase in the treated denervated muscle, but remained at about a normal level.

Other investigators, using a limited number of monkeys and not reoperating to prevent reinnervation, found that 4 weeks of galvanic stimulation started 2 weeks after denervation had only a weak retarding effect upon denervation atrophy. Another group reported that galvanic stimulation consisting of 5 contractions twice daily had no clearcut effect on denervation atrophy in dogs. Only in 6 of the 11 dogs was the atrophy slightly retarded.

In England, Gutmann and Guttmann, whose publication was considerably delayed because of the war, used a large number of rabbits with bilaterally crushed sciatic nerves and treated one side with vigorous galvanic stimulation for 20 minutes daily, including interpolated short rest periods. The strength of the stimuli was kept low enough to avoid nociceptive reactions. The effect of the therapy was evaluated by measuring the circumference of the limbs on the treated and the untreated side. The researchers concluded that galvanic exercise distinctly retards the atrophy and that, after reinnervation has started, regaining of initial muscle volume is hastened. In a second paper, the same authors reported another series of experiments, again on rabbits with both peroneal nerves sectioned and resected for some distance to prevent early nerve regeneration (later confirmed by biopsy). In yet another series, the nerves were crushed or severed and immediately sutured on both sides. Treatment was again with vigorous galvanic stimulation, but was started only 7 days after denervation. The circumferences of the legs were measured at weekly intervals, and excitability of the muscles to faradic currents determined. The spreading reflex of the toes was used as the signal of nerve regeneration. The difference in the extent of the spreading was used to compare the recovered motor function of the treated side with that of the untreated side. These experiments clearly demonstrated that the atrophy-retarding effect of the electrical treatment in animals with prevented reinnervation was greater the earlier the treatment was started. The treated muscles, in cross section, had considerably thicker muscle fibers and distinctly less connective tissue than did the control muscles. In animals with nerve regeneration, the difference between the muscles on both sides was largest at the onset of motor recovery and then declined gradually, but it was still present after 4 months. The onset of motor recovery was neither hastened nor delayed by the treatment.

Following the reported results of the animal experiments, the interest of clinicians was aroused and electrical treatment of human denervation atrophy was again advocated. In 1942, Bauwens had stated that for patients in whom motor recovery can be expected in 6 to 8 weeks, electrical treatment was probably not worthwhile, considering the needed manpower and cost.

During the next 10 to 15 years, various groups worked experimentally with animals without any major new discoveries. Solandt and coworkers treated rats from the third day after denervation for the next 11 days with the same type of stimuli but with various durations of the daily treatment sessions. Using muscle weight as the indicator of treatment results, sinusoidal currents of 25 cps gave better results than galvanic or faradic currents, or alternating currents of 60 cps. The effectiveness of treatment was increased by increasing the number of sessions from 1 to 6 per day, but the increase in the number of sessions from 3 to 6 showed only a relatively small increase in effectiveness. Lengthening the duration of the sessions from 1 to 5 minutes did not increase the effectiveness.

Reviewing the literature in 1942, the group in Chicago under Ivy found that investigators who reported treatment successes had used strong electrical stimulation, while those with more or less negative results had used weak stimulation. The importance of adjusting the stimulus used to the changing excitability of the denervated muscles was reemphasized. It was also proposed that a new machine be used that would make it easier to adapt stimulation to the varying excitability of the denervated muscles than was possible with faradic and galvanic currents. The machine was able to deliver sinusoidal currents of variable strength and frequencies from 0.1 to 500 cps. In their own experiments, the investigators were able to demonstrate that the use of a frequency of 25 cps for a denervated rat gastrocnemius was more effective than any other frequency, while for dogs a constant frequency of 3 cps was the best. For rats, 4 daily treatments of 10 minutes each gave maximal results; it was found that this treatment was more effective in respect to contractile power than to muscle weight. Stimulation for 15 seconds was as effective as stimulation for 25 minutes, while increasing the number of the daily treatments from 1 to 3 raised the effectiveness considerably; further increase in the number of sessions added very little to the effectiveness of the treatment. Six treatment sessions resulted in maximal benefit. Electrical treatment initiated after reinnervation began had no effect on the course of recovery. The effect of treatment was much less for partially denervated muscles than for completely denervated ones. In 1949, Ivy's group published a more clinical paper about its experience with electrical treatment of paralyzed muscles in patients with anterior poliomyelitis, stating that the treatment was effective as long as proper attention was paid to the excitability of the muscles and to maximal tension production during the treatment, and as long as evoking of too much pain was avoided. The treatment was even somewhat effective in poliomyelitis paralysis of very long standing, and the effect was more pronounced in respect to muscle size than to muscle power.

The investigative group in Iowa City under Hines confirmed that electrical treatment for rats, guinea pigs, and cats is effective only if considerable tension is developed during stimulation. The researchers found further that continued treatment after the onset of reinnervation is not harmful and that light volitional exercise has a favorable influence on further recovery. However, the difference after reinnervation between the treated and nontreated muscle declines the longer the treatment is continued. Moreover, they concluded that the longer the muscle length during stimulation, and the less shortening allowed to occur, the better the results.

Hill and coworkers observed after denervation of rat muscles a decrease in their oxalate and succinate metabolism during rest. This decrease was considerably diminished by daily electrical exercise of the denervated muscles.

The group under Fisher in Richmond, Virginia, established at about that time (the 1950s) that appropriate electrical treatment of denervated rabbit muscles, besides retarding the weight loss, also retarded both the loss of protein per unit muscle fiber (especially the loss of myosin) and the increase in collagen caused by the denervation. All these improvements were much enhanced when during treatment the limbs were in an extended position and the muscle contracted against a strong resistance rather than when the limbs were flexed and the muscle contracted more or less freely. In another paper Fischer's group reported that during denervation atrophy in rabbits, myoalbumin increased considerably, while myogen, soluble myosin, and an unidentified fraction of water-soluble protein decreased per unit muscle fiber. These changes are distinctly delayed by appropriate electrical treatment. Vecchioni and Tartarina confirmed in 1961 that electrical treatment can prevent the relative increase in collagen caused by denervation.

Another group under Wakin in Rochester, Minnesota, confirmed for rats essentially the findings of previous investigators, and reported that histological studies demonstrated that treated muscle fibers had fewer nuclei and larger diameters than those of untreated denervated, muscles and that 5 minutes of stimulation every 8 hours showed an optimal effect, while, at least in rats, starting the treatment only 30 days after denervation was not beneficial.

Thomas and Davenport pointed out in 1949 that in denervation atrophy the branching of intramuscular axons that had just reinnervated some muscle fibers was responsible for the then rather rapid recovery of the muscles. A few years earlier it had been well established that reinnervation of partly denervated muscle is caused mainly by sprouting of the intact residual intramuscular nerve fibers. Further investigation of this axonal sprouting and branching phenomenon revealed that it was much hastened by volitional use of the partially denervated muscle. Thus, it is likely that, in a similar way, electrical stimulation of denervated muscle begun just after the first sign of reinnervation also hastens further recovery.

Elliot and Thomson reported that denervated gastrocnemii of rats shorten more slowly and to a lesser extent than normal gastrocnemii. They showed appropriate electrical treatment of the denervated muscle under isometric conditions reverses mainly the velocity of shortening, while treatment under isotonic conditions reverses the change in the extent of shortening. Steinberger and Smith, using implanted electrodes in rabbits for 6 to 18 months, found again that the atrophy-retarding effect of electrical treatment was greatest when using maximal rectangular currents of chronaxie duration for the denervated muscles.

More recently, Herbison and coworkers reported for rats that denervated muscles treated for 30 days with strong stimulating showed in cross section an enlarged area of muscle fibers. They also reported that treatment by daily stimulating with maximal rectangular currents of 25 msec duration at 20/sec is more effective than with maximal stimulation of 100 msec duration at 2/sec. However, maximal stimulation of 0.02 msec duration at 20/sec was not effective at all.

It is astonishing that only a very small number of good clinical papers were published during and immediately after World War II. The majority of clinical papers reported observations and impressions gained from only a few patients with nerve injuries. In a large English hospital, Jackson studied the case histories and clinical findings for 92 patients with ulnar or combined median and ulnar lesions. Atrophy of the hand muscles was estimated at regular intervals by measuring hand volume by fluid displacement. Most of the patients were treated with electrical stimulation 6 times a week for 30 minutes; 90 maximal contractions were evoked by appropriate galvanic stimuli in each treatment session. The conclusions from this study were: Galvanism was of value in decreasing the rate of atrophy; its effect decreased with the time elapsed since injury; after 400 days, when there was no evidence of reinnervation, there was no beneficial effect; the treatment was beneficial in the recovery of volitional movements; treatment should begin as early as possible; and treatment is less important in children and very active youth than in adults. Liu and Lewey observed 16 patients with ulnar or median paralysis treated daily for the first month for 10 minutes and during the second month for 15 minutes with maximal sinusoidal currents, the cycles per second decreasing with the time elapsed since denervation. They measured the thickness of the hand muscles with a caliper. The treatment resulted in some increase in muscle volume, but when reinnervation occurred, the final results were no better than in comparable patients without treatment. They mentioned again the different rate of atrophy seen in different patients.

More recently, surge-faradic stimulation of the striated muscles of the pelvis was used with apparent success in a few patients with rectal incontinence, but to be beneficial the currents had to be so strong that the patients had to be anesthetized during the treatment. Despite the rather large number of papers reporting positive results with electrical treatment of denervated muscles in animals and the three reliable clinical papers, only a minority of today's neurologists favor electrical treatment of denervation palsy, while many are still or again skeptical. The main argument of the latter group is that the need in manpower and cost for adequate treatment is very high, and that when reinnervation finally occurs, even without treatment, the muscles recover satisfactorily anyway. They argue that it has not been proven yet that the final results would be better after electrical treatment. The latter argument is probably correct, provided reinnervation can occur after a few months, since many of the animal studies revealed that the longer the time after denervation, and provided reinnervation had occurred, the less the difference between the untreated muscle and the treated one. This was again confirmed in a recent study by Herbison and coworkers.

The question still remains whether or not appropriate electrical treatment of leg and foot muscles would be of value in patients with injury to the sciatic nerve high in the thigh. Nearly two and a half years will elapse before the more peripheral leg muscles and those of the foot can be reinnervated. During this long period, the fibers of these muscles would become very severely atrophied, and the connective tissues between the muscle fibers would be greatly increased. It is well known that these two conditions considerably decrease the probability of successful reinnervation. Therefore, one could expect that vigorous electrical treatment during this long period (amounting to about 700 treatment sessions) would result in larger diameters of the muscle fibers and in less connective tissue at the time of reinnervation, thus substantially increasing the probability of satisfactory reinnervation. No physician will be able to study this problem scientifically, since there are not enough patients who will agree to carry the economic burden and tolerate the prolonged unpleasant treatment. The use of large animals (e.g., dogs and goats) with the muscles of the treated and untreated side studied carefully for between 12 and 14 months could possibly give a reliable answer as to the effectiveness of treatment of denervated muscles with appropriate electrical stimulation under these conditions. Who has the patience and the economic resources to conduct such a study?

Part II

Modern Medicine
and Messages from the Past

In this section, the merits of the Hippocratic view on the art of medicine are extolled. Nature is the healer; the physician is merely the student observing and respecting its curative processes. Such respect curbs any inclination to assume control, and so the physician refrains from interfering with the homeostatic process inherent in life. Even so, Professor Schuhl appeals to the sick person to be a conscious assistant to his physician by heeding the warning voices of his own nature. Once the patient does assist, his spontaneous mind accepts responsibility for promoting the life-preserving and self-healing tendencies of the organism. The position of patient and physician changes. They become a team, partners in an active process. Schuhl also realizes that the physician has developed new and indirect ways of scrutinizing nature's secret complexities. Through advancements in scientific knowledge and technological skills, he has learned from nature how to service its vital processes, to solicit its own healing powers, and to confront the limits of both.

Common to all articles in this section is the idea that the psyche is an active participant in the healing tendencies of nature. Hippocrates could determine from the patient's physiognomy and vital processes only the course to which the patient would or would not succumb. Hippocrates was concerned exclusively with the acutely sick, and so could not rely on the alertness of the sensorium. His *Aphorisms*, which Dr. Harkins analyses in this section, were originally considered to be a textbook that students had to memorize but according to Harkins, this conception changed because of historical events. Cureau de la Chambre—a physician of such physiognomical acumen that Louis

XIV appointed him his adviser—asserted that the obvious meaning of the *Aphorisms* must be complemented by a painstaking penetration of the "hidden," "proper," and "transferred" significance. Cureau thereby enriched the heritage of antiquity by providing insight into its message. He paved the way for modern psychological and psychopathological medicine.

That different periods in medical history enrich each other reciprocally is also shown in Dr. Galdston's article on the close analogy between the "vacation" dreams of his patients and antiquity's incubation dream. The insight he gained from his psychoanalytical treatment of patients gave him insight into the experience of the ancient Greek mentality during treatment in a temple. Like Schuhl, Galdston emphasizes the common endeavor between the one in search of relief and the one contributing to it. But Galdston views less the therapeutical aspects of the endeavor. For him, the endeavor evokes from the patient deeper, more archaic sources of personality. Without such evocation and the physician's empathetic sharing of the patient's experiences, those deep, archaic sources could not be pursued, found, and interpreted. That is why Galdston recreates the religious atmosphere of the antique temple dream. He denies, however, that the interaction between patient and therapist is analogous to the temple dream in its early historical period—in which the God cures the sick person. The analogy is rather with the temple dream in its later historical period—in which the inspired temple priest is engaged in a common pursuit with the sick person. The revelatory quality of the experience and, therefore, the cure depend on the diligence of both. The dreams reported by Galdston's patients show "that the symbolism of the dream message remains the same through the ages, only the vernacular changes."

The pathography of the psychotic person described by Volmat and Signoret presents a true instance of self-healing, if we may consider as healing an adjustment the patient makes to his own satisfaction but in undisturbed contact with his social surroundings. In an unorthodox way, this patient has for some years been considered an example of mental inspiration by professionals interested in unexpected solutions to mental problems. He creates coherent artistic manifestations that unfold in autobiographical form and reveal the whole autotherapeutic procedure. The causal inner experience is revealed in all its main phases—the various attempts to reach out for gratification, the responses to deception, and the final solution, which is yet not a mental death. This patient succeeds in compelling a continual nurturing of narcissistic satisfaction through a coherent system of creation and management: He provides a glorified storage for his work; he keeps his self-portraits in his museum; he exhibits himself in symbolic terms to an audience; he turns his compulsive loquaciousness to explicatory communication with the audience about his self-centered interest; but he does not recreate traumatic starvation by making his solicitation of attention onerous. Until recently, this sick man in all likelihood would have remained a "fool" and a "madman." His efforts, which were all he had to give through the years, would not have liberated him from total isolation and cured him of estrangement from human contact. He and his art work would have remained "barren." Freud and, in his wake, the social sciences have provided the clues for interpreting the man's problem, the symbolism of his behavior and artistic communications. A qualified audience that could respond existed; so the man found physicians by proxy, and the self-healing tendency was not condemned to remain a solitary act. Isolation, an essential symptom of disease in general and of mental disease in particular, was overcome.

4

Still Physician to Oneself

At the time I was appointed lecturer at the University of Montpellier in 1936, there was much talk in the press about the manuscripts of Queen Christina, preserved at the Faculty of Medicine of this city; it was a question of offering them to Sweden, on what occasion I do not remember. So I betook myself without delay to the library to consult these manuscripts, the text of which had, incidentally, been published back in 1906.[1] I found their philosophical interest to be extremely slight if not nonexistent, as might be expected, but there was a certain psychological interest: They revealed the little that Christina had retained of the morning lessons that cost Descartes his life. It is probable that the essential thing that she learned was a saying of Tiberius, mentioned by Suetonius and afterwards by Montaigne, which Descartes cited twice: namely, that when they have passed the age of thirty, men should have "enough experience of the things that can harm or benefit them to be their own physicians."[2]

At about the same time, Lucien Lévy-Bruhl and Paul Masson-Cursel asked me to contribute to the number of the *Revue Philosophique* that they were preparing for the third centennial of the *Discours de la Méthode*, and I composed a short note entitled "Un Souvenir Cartésien dans les Pensées de la Reine Christine (A Cartesian Bequest in the Thoughts of Queen Christina)." It appeared in 1937 (pp. 368–369).

Some twenty years later, when I was preparing an anthology of *Etudes Platoniçiennes* (Paris, 1960), I included this study in it under the title "Le Médecin de Soi-Même: de Socrate à la Reine Christine" (pp. 166–171). I expanded it slightly, showing how, in seeking the origin of this saying, it is necessary to go back to the famous precept of Apollo at Delphi—commented upon by Socrates in the *Memorabilia* (IV, 7, 9) in a medical perspective and then to come down again "from Socrates to Tiberius, from Tiberius by Suetonius to Montaigne and to Descartes, and finally, to the queen of Sweden" (p. 171).

On the advice of M. Canguilhem, Mme Evelyn Aziza Shuster took up the study of this theme again some years ago, going into it more thoroughly, in a little volume published in 1973, which is her doctoral dissertation, defended in 1970. The first three chapters, which compose the first part, take up the three principal stages that we have mentioned so far:

1. Descartes wished to form a mechanical biology permitting effective therapeutics. But difficulties accumulated, and Descartes admitted that, as M. Gueroult expressed it, "The human body is not merely pure extension, but also psycho-physical substance."[3] The result is that "understanding must give way to feeling, the only justified instrument for true knowledge of life."[4]

The voice of feeling is that of nature—of the "inner physician." We must know how to listen to it, to let it restore us spontaneously rather than resort to drugs and to those bleedings that were to kill Descartes at Stockholm.

2. Descartes had read Montaigne, who placed confidence in instinct, not in physicians "who make health sick."[5] "Whatever I take that is disagreeable to me does me harm, and nothing harms me that I do hungrily and gladly."[6]

3. Nature, says a famous and often-cited text of Hippocrates,[7] is the patient's physician. "The role of the physician," Mme Shuster goes on to say, "is to foresee the course and the outcome of the disease rather than to intervene" (p. 33); he should respect the "regulating spontaneity of organic life" (p. 34). This principle is "the basis of the theme of physician to oneself" (p. 35).

As far as Plato is concerned, I think that it would be well to introduce here a text from the *Timaeus* (p. 89b–d), where it is pointed out that just as living beings are born with a certain span of existence assigned them by destiny, so diseases have a certain duration. If one tries to shorten that by means of drugs, one runs the risk of aggravating the disease. What is needed is an appropriate regimen, not an irritating pharmacopoeia.[8]

This is a Hippocratic idea as well, and one that is being revived in our day with the work of Professor Nicolle on the duration and extent of certain diseases. The reader of the *Timaeus* was quite naturally inclined to prefer the regimen that he had been led to establish for himself to the pharmacopoeia of the physicians. Let us add that treatises on regimen were in fashion at that time; they showed how it was necessary to vary it according to the seasons, climates, and circumstances; for example, one of the greatest successors of Hippocrates, Diocles Carystius, had written a regimen at the request of a king of Macedonia. What has come down to us from it has been well studied and presented by Wilamovitz in an excellent book.[9]

The second part of Mme Shuster's work presents new and generally little-known facts about the notion of "physician to oneself" among the different authors of the seventeenth and eighteenth centuries.

Jean Devaux (1649-1729) published in 1682 at Leyden a book entitled *Le Médecin de Soi-Même, ou l'Art de Recouvrir la Santé par l'Instinct.*[10] He gives as example the country folk, who "by no means go to a druggist for oriental leaves, senna from the Levant ... at excessive price."[11] Another example is animals, whose instinct suffices to keep them in health; the Stoics had already noted it; they attributed to animals a certain discernment, which Descartes did not grant them, but which Cureau de la Chambre claimed for them in his *Traité de la Connaissance des Animaux,* published in 1648. La Fontaine's marvelous *Discours à Madame de la Sablière* should also be cited here.

"The patient, when a prey to disease, has little control of himself and loses his memory for the cure of his illness," one reads in a *Régime de Santé,* published in 1686 under the name of De La Cour, who in addition was opposed to "bleedings and purgations."

In 1692, there also was published in Paris a work by a certain Flamant: *L'Art de se Conserver La Santé ou le Médecin de Soi-Même,* which recommends a prudent moderation in the use of remedies. Flamant and Devaux were to be translated into German in 1721. But Leibnitz had already read Devaux in 1701; citing him, he wrote at that time (to Sackenholz) that we have lost natural instinct "by an artificial way of life."

In London, J. Archer published in 1673 *Everyman, His Own Doctor,* in which he tells his reader to know his constitution before going to consult the physician.

At the University of Halle, founded in 1693, there was for more than twenty years a conflict between two well-known physicians: Hoffmann, a mechanist, and Stahl, an animist. Both ended as naturists.

Stahl (1660–1734) was called to Halle in 1694 by Hoffmann (1660–1742). He attributes the organic finality of living being to the action of a rational principle, a reasonable mind.[12] Only exceptional cases "need the intervention of medical technique."

A pupil of Stahl, Berghauer, in 1707 defended at Halle a doctoral dissertation entitled *De Medicina sine Medico*, which advocated submission to nature. In 1696, another dissertation had been defended by J. A. Lassius: *De Autocratia Naturae sive Spontanea Morborum Excressione et Convalescentia*, which required the physician to be *physicodidascalus*.

For Hoffmann, however, the vital principle is found in matter— an active matter, endowed with force—which does not prevent him from referring to Hippocrates and publishing two dissertations, one entitled *De Natura Morborum Medicatrice Mechanica* (1699) and the other, *De Medico Sui Ipsius* (1704). Excerpts from these are found in the appendix to Mme Shuster's book (pp. 141–149). He advises us to observe a regimen in harmony with nature and an art of living according to reasonable rules; to avoid excess, abrupt changes, melancholy; to seek pure air, to choose foods that agree with us and are proportionate to our exercise; to shun charlatans and violent persons.

In Verona, Joseph Gazola (1661–1715) wrote *Il Mondo Ingannato da Falsi Medici* (Prague, 1719), translated into French at Leyden in 1735 under the title *Préservation contre la Charlatanerie des Faux Médicins*. He affirms that "it is better to do without a physician than not to have a good one." He refers to Malebranche, who had not lost confidence in the value of the senses and who compared the activity of the physician, as concerned health, to that of the spiritual adviser for salvation: Both should act with discrimination.

Finally, among the works of Linnaeus is found a thesis, *Medicus Sui Ipsius* (Upsala, 1768). Attributed to J. Grisselius, it sums up Linnean dietetics, which does not overlook the pleasure of change: *variatio delectat*. The importance of hygiene is found emphasized again in Kant's *Conflit des Facultés* (1798; Gibelin translation, 1935).

The third part of Mme Shuster's book is entitled "La Fin d'un Mythe et son Interprétation."

For Condorcet (a pupil of Tronchin), healing nature is a myth (he of course does not use the word); he knows the works of Lavoisier and his sketch of a theory of organic regulations (*Mémoires sur la Respiration des Animaux, sur la Transpiration des Animaux*). For him "nature is a system of regulators" (p. 98). She "speaks only if one questions her (p. 99); let us add that Bacon had already been attempting to subject her to interrogation— a thing that the patient cannot do. But Zimmermann remains faithful to the old ideas in his *Traité de l'Expérience* (1763–1767), translated in 1774, republished in 1792.

At the end of the eighteenth century and during the nineteenth century there appeared a whole series of treatises on domestic and popular medicine. Some of their authors were Hecquet (1661–1737); Riond (1842), *La Médecine Populaire ou l'Art de Guérir Indiqué par la Nature;* Morel de Rubempré (1826), *Véritable Médecine sans Médecin* and *Le Médecin de Vénus ou l'Art de se Guérir Soi-Même* (1895).

The most famous, as well as the most popular, was Raspail (1794–1878), whose panacea was camphor, as coal tar was Berkeley's.

During this time, pathology and therapeutics were taking giant steps forward. Nevertheless, Charcot, in his admission thesis, speaks in praise of *"expectation in medicine."* Béchaud and Axenfeld in their report on the progress of medicine in France for the Exposition of 1867 (the same series in which Revaisson discussed philosophy) praised the daring of the pharmacopoeia, while recognizing that "to allow to recover is one of the conquests of contemporary medicine" (p. 68, cited p. 118).

Claude Bernard himself emphasized the importance of the regulatory mechanisms, which assure the constancy of the internal milieu; Cannon, in turn, in the twentieth century, speaks of the "homeostasis" that constitutes what he calls "the wisdom of the body,"[13] and gives cicatrization as an example of "self-repair." Thus, after all, the notion of *vis reparatrix* is found justified at the same time that it is possible to determine its limits: Nothing can replace insulin for the diabetic.

Meanwhile, a certain number of homeostatic reflex devices had been discovered: the depressor nerve of the heart in 1867, the carotid sinus in 1924 (p. 122). But organic spontaneity can exceed therapeutics (anaphylaxis, histamine).

"In exposing the disorders of adaptation, under which one can group together all the phenomena of anaphylaxis, allergy, hyperactivity of the organism, modern medicine reveals, at the very root of life, a possibility of aberration that limits, sometimes cruelly, its wisdom" (p. 123); "but should not the very concept of regulation comprise in its definition that of the eventual insufficiency of its capacities?" (p. 126).

Therefore, it seems difficult, as Mme Shuster points out in her conclusion (p. 135), to proclaim "individual self-sufficiency in the regulation of organic human life."

And yet, is nothing to be retained of the thought of Tiberius repeated by Descartes?

Certainly, it is indispensable for the physician to intervene, and intervene as soon as possible, in time to treat cancer, lung edema, infarction. But this is no reason to reject everything that the notion of "physician to oneself" implies. Like the slave doctors of whom Plato spoke, today's physicians are often hard pressed, more than those of the preceding generation, and have not much time to give to the "single colloquy" dear to Duhamel. It is good for the patient to know and be able to tell what his allergies, his intolerances are; whether or not, for example, he can stand a certain medicinal cocktail. The new chemical pharmacopoeia works wonders, but sometimes, for lack of sufficient experimentation, holds surprises; and I very much like the prudence of those old physicians who gave preference to proven drugs of long standing and whose experienced clinical glance detected at first sight what laboratory examinations reveal today, but did it more humanely. "Do you wish to treat your patient, or make a doctor of him?" Plato asked a free-men's physician, who was explaining to his patient what his condition was. But an illness understood is often already somewhat cured: "The patient," said Ducuing, "is never wrong." And, in fact, it is he who knows where he suffers, if he does not know from what. And he sometimes knows what he cannot tolerate: Penicillin, for instance, can expose certain persons to the risk of shock, if the physician is not warned. The family doctor knew all that, but the doctor in the dispensary stands every chance of not knowing it, if he is not put on guard. This is why it is advisable still to remain something of a "physician to oneself."

REFERENCES

1. Edition de Bilt, Stockholm: I. *L'ouvrage du loisir*. II. *Les sentiments*.
2. Au Marquis de Newcastle, Oct. 1645; *Entretiens Avec Burman*, A. J. IV, 329, and V, 178.
3. *Descartes selon l'Ordre des Raisons, l'Ame et Corps*. Paris, Aubier, 1953, II, Chapter XX, p. 248, p. 13, n. 4.
4. l.c., pp. 242–246.
5. *Essais* (Pléiade), II, Chapter 37, p. 857.
6. l.c., III, Chapter 13, p. 1220.
7. *Epidémies*, VI, Ch. 5, 315, p. 51, n.
8. Cf. *My Fabulation Platonicienne*. 2nd edition, 1968, p. 111.
9. U. von Wilamovitz, Moellendorf F.: *Diokles von Karystos, die griechische Medizin und die Schule des Aristoteles*, Berlin, 1938.
10. *Facsimilés* pl. I, p. 89.
11. Jean Devaux, l.c., p. 88; cited p. 48, no. 2.
12. A reference to remember: F. Courtès. *La Raison et la Vie Scientifique et l'Idéologie en Allemagne de la Reforme jusqu'a Kant*. 1972.
13. Cannon, Walter Bradford: *The Wisdom of the Body*. New York, 1932. French translation 1939 (p. 120, no. 6).

Paul W. Harkins

5

Cureau de la Chambre
and Hippocrates' *Aphorisms*

"Life is short, the Art long." With this pithy, proverbial sentence, Hippocrates opens the first of the seven sections of his *Aphorisms*. But his statement seems only partly true, since the art he mentions is the art of medicine, and the life is that which is so often saved and prolonged by the physician's skill. And the art of medicine has had but a brief existence in modern times when one considers the recent explosions of medical knowledge, the incredible new surgical procedures, the wonder drugs made available to the clinician by research, and the abatement and even eradication of what were once common and deadly diseases.

One does not have to go too far back in the history of medicine to come to a day when a diagnosis could not be confirmed by laboratory tests, EKGs, and other sophisticated devices. Before that day, the art was long because it extended back through the ages to some five centuries before Christ, when medicine emerged from magic to become rational and scientific. Hippocrates (b. 460 B.C.) was perhaps the first to reject the notion that human ills were punishments sent by the gods to men. Rightly called "the Father of Medicine," he was the first to maintain that every disease has its own nature and arises from external causes. He had no stethoscope, no thermometer, and no X-rays, yet his skill of observation and reasoning and his insight into symptoms gave him great powers of diagnosis and prognosis.

Although his clinic was attached to a temple on the Greek island of Cos (a sanctuary to which patients came seeking cures by such superstitious means as the cult of incubation), his treatment of disease looked mainly to a natural cure[1] and made minimal use of the primitive drugs available to him. He also saw clearly the effects of diet and environment on health, and left us a book that amounts to a treatise on human ecology: *On Air, Waters, and Localities.*

In fact, some seventy-two works on medicine are attributed to Hippocrates, although the majority of these would seem to be works of his students—perhaps notes made by them at their master's lectures. Some of these, most notably the *Aphorisms,* continued to be used as textbooks by medical students up to the nineteenth century. It is not strange, therefore, that through the ages, professors of medicine were always seeking new insights and explications of the *Aphorisms.* This brief study will present one such explication by summarizing the method used and offering several examples from a Latin work published by M. Cureau de la Chambre (1594–1669), entitled *Novae Methodi pro Explanandis Hippocrates & Aristotle Specimen* (Paris, 1655).

A physician to Louis XIV, de la Chambre acquired a great reputation in such varied fields as belles lettres, philosophy, and medicine. That he deserved this reputation is clear from this work, which deals with Hippocrates, the physician, and Aristotle, the philosopher, and also offers a new method for explicating the *Aphorisms* of the former and the *Physics* of the latter.[2]

The book is truly a *specimen,* or example, since it is what might be called a trial balloon offered by Cureau to his fellow physicians of the School of Paris so that his method might benefit from his colleagues' judgment or, if need be, their correction. Since it is merely a specimen, Cureau takes only section II of the *Aphorisms* to exemplify his method; explanations of the remaining six sections are promised for a later date if the specimen is successful.[3]

Why should the aphorisms need explication at all, much less a new method? One must remember that when they were composed, medicine was just emerging from magic and religion. Earlier works were written in terse and oracular language; the aphorisms do not entirely defy this tradition.

For de la Chambre there were other reasons. Everywhere, he says, new principles of nature (perhaps under Cartesian influence) and new systems of healing are being proposed.[4] These, of course, are good as long as they do not reject the dogmas of ancient wisdom on the pretext that these are brief to the point of obscurity. The aphorisms are oracular in style, but Cureau promises that his method will free them from all darkness and, through a process of inference, make clear what may by itself be obscure. He will bring newness to the old, splendor to what has fallen into neglect. Furthermore, where several passages have become textually corrupted, he will restore to these places their true meaning.

In the course of his deliberations Cureau discovered that he must look for three things in the *Aphorisms:* the meaning of each aphorism and the application to which it can be directed; the basis on which it rests; and whether their distribution and arrangement is based on a particular plan.

The meaning of the words has often been obscured either by textual corruptions, by the use of words that sound alike but differ in meaning, or by involved sentence structure. Furthermore, Cureau often finds one meaning in the literal statement of an aphorism and another in its application. And at times the application does not become immediately clear through the words of the aphorism, so that it is in the application that the true and principal meaning of the aphorism must be sought.

The physician should take special pains to discover the meaning of a given aphorism, since they are all directed toward a practical application—be it in the area of prognosis or therapy. There also usually is another meaning that is not clearly expressed and that Cureau calls the hidden meaning; this may be either "proper" or "transferred" or both. He distinguishes these meanings by saying that the hidden proper meaning comes close to the matter expressed by the aphorism's wording, whereas the hidden transferred meaning is directed to other but similar matters.

Cureau exemplifies this by citing *Aphorism* II.1, "A disease in which sleep causes distress is a deadly disease," where he finds the meaning in the applications. The evident application is the prognosis of a distressed sleep; the hidden proper application has to do with the cure of this symptom; the hidden transferred application extends to other things which resemble a distress-causing sleep.

Hippocrates hardly ever presents the basis on which any of the aphorisms rests. Cureau attributes this omission to the fact that Hippocrates was striving for a brevity suited to memorization by medical students, and furthermore was trying to give his precepts on medicine a quasi-legal binding force that would command rather than persuade. As an explicator, Cureau considers it his function to investigate and explain the basis for the order and arrangement of the aphorisms.

In Cureau's day, two theories on the order and arrangement of the *Aphorisms* existed: One held that they were arranged in a fixed and invariable series; the other held that there was no order but that, like Sibylline oracles written on leaves, the aphorisms were scattered helter-skelter at the whim of chance. Cureau finds neither theory totally acceptable but feels that, at least in Hippocrates' mind, each aphorism has some connection with the preceding one, at least on the basis of similarity.

Cureau admits that his inquiry into the order and arrangement of the aphorisms has little to do with medical practice, but he feels that it has added some new understanding to the collection. In investigating the applications, he has not only restored corrupted passages but also confirmed others by discovering new proofs for them.

Both Hippocrates and Cureau realized that for treatment to be rational it must have a theoretical basis. For both of them this basis was the theory of the four cardinal fluids or humors: blood, phlegm, yellow bile, and black bile. Harmonious blending of these humors produced health; disharmony of the humors resulted in sickness; innate heat (greatest in youth but declining with age) was a determinant of health. Disease had to be treated by rectifying any disharmony of the humors, which have a natural tendency to equilibrium and are likely to regain that state through the healing power of nature. My translations of Cureau's explications of three Hippocratic aphorisms (Section II— numbers, 1, 4, and 5) should serve to support this thesis and to illustrate de la Chambre's new method of explication.

Aphorism II.1

A disease in which sleep causes distress is a deadly one; but if sleep is beneficial, the disease is not deadly.

Meaning of the Aphorism

Not every distressful sleep is deadly, but only that which causes serious and frequent affliction, and brings on torpidity, or convulsion, or extreme sluggishness, or some other ruinous symptom. Even though it increases fever, or provokes thirst, or causes some other vexation, sleep is not necessarily deadly, but should be considered bad. Apparently Hippocrates here either used "deadly" in the sense of "bad," as he has done in other places, or wished the less serious to be included in the more serious—as if to say that it is always bad if sleep causes affliction, but it is deadly if it causes serious affliction. Thus, when he said that to derive benefit from sleep is "not deadly," he meant to say it is "good and not bad." As regards a sleep that affords benefit, one kind is good and conducive to health, another is by no means bad but has no influence on health. Hence, he did not consider what is good and healthful to be the opposite of what is deadly; for not every healthful thing is a thing which is not deadly, nor is every good a thing which brings no bad.

Basis of the Aphorism

Distressful sleep, however, is bad, both as a sign and as a cause. It indicates that an abundant and perverse rising of a humor is being carried to the head, and that the natural warmth gathered therein is unable to overcome the disease-producing causes. It also threatens new ills when it brings on either torpidity or delirium, increases internal inflammations, produces paroxysms and symptoms which last longer than usual and, least important, when it deprives the patient of the benefit of wakefulness.

Evident Application and Order of the Aphorism

This aphorism seems to be limited to prognosis and only to that prognosis which is derived from the condition of sleep in cases of acute fevers. (It is unlikely that Hippocrates spoke of these diseases throughout the preceding book, and, looking ahead to the symptoms of these ailments, began with sleep as the more obvious symptom which always accompanies them.) However, he often included many other meanings in each precept and directed the individual aphorisms toward more applications than words can describe. Hence, he describes sleep here in such a way that one not only can judge the nature of acute fevers but can also draw a similar inference for other diseases. For if sleep is harmful or beneficial in these other ailments, it indicates the same prognosis as in acute fevers. If a torpid or disturbed sleep has come upon a patient in a long-continued ailment, it should arouse no less apprehension than it does in an acute illness; even in healthy people, it is an indication that diseases are very close at hand, as Hippocrates has explained in his book on dreams (*De Insominiis*).

Hidden Proper Application

By his prognosis Hippocrates leads us directly to the therapy. He hints that we must keep in check the sleep which brings on distress, whether it is caused by disease or by nature. We must curb the sleep which occurs contrary to nature as, for instance, in ailments marked by lethargy and at the onset of paroxysms. In cataphoric cases such sleep often embraces the whole force of the evil; in paroxysms it augments the duration and slows down nature's movement to a crisis[5] because it keeps within the body all the soot-like refuse which wakefulness would sift through the pores of the skin. In pestilential diseases, however, we must also curb the sleep that comes according to nature, because it retains in the body the diseased matter which should be cast out. This applies to internal inflammations which are irritated by sleep because warmth gathers inside the body and the humors are driven to the focus of the disease; it also applies to cases of catarrh and catarrhal discharge because sleep gathers the humors in the brain where they foster and increase ailments of this sort. Although sleep should not be altogether prevented in the above-mentioned diseases, we must limit it to the amount needed to sustain the patient's strength. Not only must we prevent a sleep that comes on contrary to nature but we must also use suitable remedies to rout the causes which produce this sleep.

Transferred Applications

By discussing one species Hippocrates deals with the entire class, for under the heading of sleep he includes everything else that ought to benefit patients but still brings them distress. For it is a universal axiom that a thing is deadly if it combines an increase in evil with something from which the greatest good is expected. Therefore, if anything within or outside of the body brings distress to the patient while it should ease his pain, it signals danger just as sleep does. If the cutting of a vein, for instance, exasperates a disease, it proves that nature is incapacitated, or happens to be busy elsewhere, or that the ballast of humors has been disturbed by the disease and been transferred to superior portions (of the body). If purging is the basis for the complaint, it proves that nature was not equal to the remedy, or that undigested matter has been stirred up in a reversal of the usual order, with the result that the diseases break out anew and the symptoms increase. The same principle applies to food. If it is taken properly yet destroys the strength it should preserve or restore, nature is either undone or weakened by a superfluity of bad humors. All these things also have a bearing on judgment, but do not make judgment. Consequently, we must say the same about them as about a sleep which causes distress; and it is true that a disease in which sweats or other critical upheavals cause distress is a deadly one.

Aphorism II.4

Neither repletion, nor fasting, nor anything else is good when it is more than natural.

Order and Arrangement of the Aphorism

Excess in sleep and sleeplessness easily leads to excess in other things.

Hippocrates did not state this as an aphorism because, as is commonly held, he wished the preceding Aphorism[6] to be confirmed by new examples.

Meaning of the Aphorism

He wanted to point out that among the things that exceed the limits imposed by nature, some, like sleep and sleeplessness, are bad while others, like fasting and repletion, are not good. Sleep and sleeplessness are always bad when they are excessive; fasting and repletion are sometimes bad and sometimes not bad, but they are never good. Although an aversion against food or an excessive appetite during a fever are never good, they often do no harm and are counted among the signs of irregularity. Intoxication in healthy persons should never be praised; while it is sometimes harmless, it often invites disease.

Application of the Aphorism

Hippocrates aimed this aphorism primarily at acute fevers, as if he wished to teach us that in such fevers everything that is more than natural should be avoided, especially when disease is imminent or nature is beginning some work. What is more than natural oppresses nature. Furthermore, if nature is already subject to an affliction and a new trouble is added, it collapses under a burden which it is not equal to bearing.

Hidden Application

There is no doubt that Hippocrates directed the application of this aphorism also toward many other things. For there is nothing designed to preserve or restore health which is not subject to this law of something that is more than natural. But keen talent is needed to weigh carefully what constitutes each individual's proper nature and what is more than natural. Hippocrates wished nutriment to be "equal to equal"; thus (in the seventh Aphorism[7]), he prescribed wine drunk "equal to equal," as a remedy for distress, yawning, and shivering, which did not mean wine mixed with an equal portion of water, as Galen thought, but wine proportionate to temperament, habit, season, etc. Hippocrates already, in an earlier aphorism,[8] had mentioned that we must take season, district, age, and habit into account. He looked for equality in all things, an equality which considers nature and strength. For equality is being according to nature; anything that is more than natural is unequal and harmful.

One may rightly ask whether any rule can be given for recognizing and linking together proportionate equality and moderation.

There can be; otherwise medicine which orders this equality of proportion to be used in all things would be empty and blind. But we cannot establish a rule which embraces all topics in which such equality is desirable, nor a rule which will let us recognize that equality by a method which will never mislead us. Since we must follow one rule of equality of proportion in the case of health and another in the case of disease, and since the rule that applies to foods, for example, does not apply to exercise, equality of proportion cannot be defined by a single means of measurement. If it could, it would mean that not only the quantity of medical remedies but also the quality, manner and reason for using them would be the same for the personal nature of each individual man. However, the physician does not cure mankind; he cures Socrates.[9] This is a difficult task and, if we had to decide on a remedy that is applicable to all cases, we would not find one since there is no science of individual things.

Many have indeed tried to establish a norm of moderation for certain groups of things. For food it consists, for example, of never taking more than is desired, as Avicenna would have it; or of always taking less than is desired, as Hippocrates wished; or, of taking only as much as can be digested, according to Celsus. But norms like these are truncated and misleading. They pertain only to the temperate man and delimit only the quantity of food, while we must show equal care for moderation in the quality of food. The bilious person is certainly harmed if he takes less than he desires; the melancholic person is hurt if he takes as much as he desires; in addition, many of the things which are easily digested prove to be harmful.

Moderation in exercise, which has been defined in terms of weariness beyond fatigue and copious perspiration, is subject to the same difficulties, for it too considers only temperate man. But exercise should be increased in the case of apathetic or phlegmatic people and decreased for those who have an excess of bile; very little exercise and often none at all is indicated for those weakened by age or disease. The same method applies to all other things necessary for living, for what is moderate in these matters can hardly be stated in a universal law.

And if any law comes close to that point, it is the law which is based on the sense of well-being [*euphoria*]. For it stands to reason that things which are beneficial and easily tolerated are proportioned, equal, and appropriate to nature. There is nothing which promotes good health, nor any condition of life, to which this rule does not apply since it pertains to food, air, love, medicines, temperaments, humors, and all other matters both natural and not in accord with nature; this rule holds good for the young and the old, for any temperament, for the healthy and the sick; hence, Hippocrates wanted it to be the sole measure of the benefit of remedies in these cases.

However, we cannot always trust this rule since habit often leads us astray. Things to which we have become accustomed, for instance, even though they are bad, are more easily tolerated than the good things to which we have not become used (as is noted in the fiftieth Aphorism[10] of section II), or they corrupt nature and bring on disease. Often, too, a corrupted appetite desires what is bad and, for a period of time, easily tolerates things which will result in destruction. We must therefore be mindful of that very exact prudence which considers all possibilities and reduces general precepts to individual conditions and the proper nature of each person.

Aphorism II.5

Spontaneous weariness indicates disease.

Order and Arrangement of the Aphorism

After a precept on things which are more than natural, there follows readily the thought of spontaneous weariness resulting from more than natural humors.

Meaning and Basis of the Aphorism

If these humors are at fault because of their quantity, then the result is a tensive [tensiva] weariness; if, however, their quality is at fault, then the result is ulcerative weariness; if the trouble lies with both the quantity and the quality of the humors, then the result is a phlegmonous weariness due to an inflamation under the skin. All these results indicate diseases because they point to a plethora or superfluity of bad humors which cause almost all diseases. Tensive weariness passes easily into apoplexy because the passages are stopped up, or into malignant fever because the blood has been corrupted. Ulcerative weariness causes either ulcers or arthritis when the bile remains fixed in the joints, fever when the bile runs back into the veins, and colic when it returns to the intestines. Phlegmonous weariness is the worst of all and quickly develops into the most acute fever.

Hidden Application

Although this prognosis is limited to spontaneous weariness, it can also be extended to the weariness that follows bodily activities. If someone, after light work, for instance, falls into ulcerative or phlegmonous weariness, there is a well-justified fear that he may fall ill because his body seems to harbor a considerable superfluity of bad humors which has given rise to these symptoms after only a slight effort. There is no doubt then that this is not a case of spontaneous weariness but that the origin is the same and the disease itself as dangerous as spontaneous weariness.

Transferred Application

But we must not limit this aphorism to weariness alone. Hippocrates includes in this one category all other spontaneous affections which are based on an underlying superfluity of bad humors, dispositions which indicate that illnesses will soon appear. To this category belongs any unusual bodily change, better or worse, as, for instance, when the body becomes fuller or withers away, when it shines forth with a more florid complexion or turns pale, when it is oppressed by a sleep that is too heavy or is wasted by sleeplessness; when it is painful to turn the eyes and when the veins are bent and throbbing, when there is frequent shivering, or sweating, or yawning, or when breathing becomes feeble and the senses become dull. And then there are the dreams that Hippocrates noted, called *synesian,* i.e., proper to each individual, through which a person can gain some perception of his future diseases.

Proper Application

Since all these conditions indicate diseases, it behooves us to remove their causes and to do so by rather strong remedies if the threatened disease is serious. But if we are prevented from using these remedies or if the affection seems less serious, we must overcome it by a suitable diet. Although it may appear to the ordinary person that the art of medicine uses only the more severe remedies to protect a person's health, this is not the case; it often employs milder ones because it is well aware that nature preserves nature. Hippocrates proved the latter in his excellent book *On Dreams,* (*De Insomniis*) where he attempts to cure any diseases which threaten by prescribing a diet and nothing else—except in two or three instances where he prescribed hellebore.

REFERENCES

1. To him is attributed the doctrine of "nature as the healer of diseases," the *vis medicatrix naturae* of the later Latin writers and of today.
2. Dr. W. Riese, in his monograph, "La théorie des passions à la lumière de la pensée médicale du XVIIᵉ siècle," a supplement to *Confinia*

Psychiatrica 8 (1965), devotes two chapters (pp. 19–44) to Cureau de la Chambre's treatment of the passions, which reflects the contribution of both a physician and a philosopher.

3. The *Catalogue Générale* of the Bibliothèque Nationale in Paris lists copies of three printings of the *Specimen*, 1655, 1662, and 1668 (the year before Cureau's death). There is no mention of any work explicating all seven sections of the *Aphorisms*. Perhaps this argument from silence may indicate that the *Specimen* merited reprinting but not enlargement and completion.

4. Dominant factors in seventeenth-century medicine were Harvey's discovery of the circulation of the blood (published in 1628), the mechanical philosophy of Descartes, the contemporary progress of physics, the introduction of chemical explanations of morbid processes, and the rise of the spirit of inquiry and innovation so characteristic of the scientific movement.

5. Hippocrates called the process by which the humors came into harmony *pepsis* (Latin *coctio*), which was later elaborated as a series of "digestions." The turning point at which *pepsis* is complete is the *crisis*, a term that still bears some of its original medical meaning. The crisis was expected on certain days.

6. *Aphorisms* II.3 reads: "Sleep or sleeplessness in undue measure are both bad."

7. Cureau must mean *Aphorisms* VII.56, which reads: "Distress, yawning, and shivering are removed by drinking wine equal to equal."

8. *Aphorisms* I.17 reads (although the text is uncertain): "To some food should be given once, to others twice; in greater quantity or less, a little at a time. Something too must be conceded to season, locality, habit, and age."

9. That is, an individual man.

10. *Aphorisms* II.50 reads: "Things to which one has long been accustomed, even though they be more severe than unaccustomed things, usually cause less distress. . . ."

Iago Galdston

6

The Incubation Dream:
Its Modern Equivalent

*Changing times bring about certain alternations in views
and significance but the meanings and their effect remain
essentially the same.*

—C. A. Meier

The Incubation Dream, historically defined, is singular in circumstance
and occasion. It is no ordinary dream, but rather a dream dreamt in
a consecrated setting by one who is ailing and who has come to sup-
plicate the indwelling god to cure him of his illness. It is, in other
words, a dream that embodies both medical and religious elements.
According to Mary Hamilton, "Supplicants approached the god by
sacrifices and performance of rites best calculated to win his favor,
and then in the place most likely to be visited by the deity, either
temple, or the appointed sleeping hall, lay down to sleep awaiting a
divine visitation."[1]

The rites of incubation were practiced in numerous places, and
the gods whose favors were solicited were many. The most famous
among them was Asclepius—initially, like the other gods, a chthonian
deity, that is, a hero who had gone down into the earth, and who had
gained from the earth both the power of sending dreams and the
gifts of healing.

The myths about the genesis of Asclepius and his ascendency
to divinity are far too complicated to treat in this brief presentation.
We can accept Asclepius, as he is historically represented, his temples
(the most famous among them those at Trika, Cos, and Epidaurus),
and the known data on the practice of incubation in the temples'
abaton, that is, dormitory. We will take note of the little that is known

of the initial or preparatory rituals and ceremonies, the sacrifices and rites of purification that were practiced in the Asclepian temples. They were, we are told, practiced in good faith, and with dignity, in a setting that was inspiring.

Our concern is with the ultimate, the incubation dream. What was its nature, and how, if at all, was it effective? Perhaps it is best to distinguish between, and thus separate, incubation and the dream. Incubation was the act, after appropriate religious preparations, of going to sleep in the consecrated locus. Incubation is thus, as the German word describes it, *Tempelschlaf*. The dream is a matter apart. It would or would not come, and historically it could come in many shapes and forms.[2]

In earlier times, it was more of a visitation than a dream. The god appeared in person and effected the cure. The sixteenth testimonial on Stele I, found at Epidaurus, reads as follows: "Euhippus had had for six years the point of a spear in his jaw. As he was sleeping in the temple, the god extracted the spearhead and gave it into his hands. Euhippus departed cured, and he held the spearhead in his hands."[3]

In the testimonies inscribed on the Epidaurus Stelae, the god enucleated eyes and reimplanted them; he mended a broken goblet to spare the servant from the wrath of his master; he cured a man of his baldness; he relieved women of their sterility and brought on the long-delayed birth of offspring.[4] In all this Asclepius was in effect, or so it would appear, for some of the testimonies bespeak the rational rather than the miraculous, a miracle worker.

But that was in the earlier days of the Asclepian cult, before the times of the Roman Caesars.

Mary Hamilton, citing Karvadias, distinguishes two separate periods in the Asclepian cult at Epidaurus: the first, when the god cured the supplicant in person and miraculously, and the second, later period, when the god gave the patient guidance in dreams.[5]

> The treatment is still by temple sleep, but now the god does not serve by personal intervention. He rather points the way to salvation. Dreams were sent and tokens given to the supplicant and an interpretation of these had then to be made. According to the interpretation, the patient pursued what in many cases appears to have been a long and tedious cure. The simplicity and reassuring certainty of the ancient inscriptions had disappeared, and instead of all being righted by the laying-on of a healing hand, the patient had to follow out carefully a course of treatment and submit to a strict regime.[6]

It is this order of dream, the interpretation of which guided the treatment of the patient, that is my particular concern, though the earlier, miraculous dream interests me little less. The difference is that I have had *some* experience with the former, and but little if any with the miracle dream. Yet scanning the dreams and the resulting cures of the earlier period, they seems to me little more miraculous—that is, incomprehensible and inexplicable—than I find any cure to be. In modern medicine, the little we know obscures the vast unknown. Every cure has in it much that is miraculous, be the cure effected by means of an antitoxin, an antibiotic, or a chemotherapeutic agent. For all the accumulated lore in this realm of knowledge, most mysterious and miraculous I find the effects, notably the therapeutic ones, that one personality can produce in another. However, I do not intend to re-argue once again what has been argued so many times before, to wit, the meaning and authenticity of the miracle working dreams. The Edelsteins, in their splendid and authoritative study on Asclepius, have canvassed the pros and cons of this controversy and I gladly rest on and concur with their summating sentences:

> Unless it is simply true that the gods in ancient times performed miracles and only left this world of ours, as of old did justice, that loathe that race of men and fly heavenward; there are good reasons for the success which nature and the experience of the supplicants brought about in the temples of Asclepius.[7]

They also write: "The miracle, that is, the recovery of one whom 'the doctor has to admit that only a miracle can save him— *such* a miracle sometimes happens. Men of today ascribe it to nature; men of antiquity ascribed it to the deity." Can it not be that nature includes "the deity"?

Here I must leave the miracle-working dream and turn to what has been aptly named the therapeutic dream, and here, too, I must change the historian's hat for that of the clinician, the psychotherapist, and speak of my more intimate experiences.

My interest in the incubation dream derives from my experiences with what I have come to call "the vacation dream." Some years ago I observed that I myself, when on vacation, and most notably when abroad, that is, distant from my accustomed environment and far from my common preoccupations, dreamt uncommon dreams. They were uncommon in that they were more intensively experienced, reached further back in my life, and touched on matters and issues that related to the very core of my being—to my long-dead father, for example, and to issues of my distant past.

These dreams troubled me a little, but puzzled me much. I am accustomed to confronting the emergence of my unconscious. But why the intensity and the uncommon depth, and mostly, why dreamt when on vacation and not during everyday life? I ventured some explanations, but found them unsatisfying. The problem remained with me, and I mulled it over and over. Then in time I perceived that my patients, too—not all of them, but a goodly number—had dreamt singularly deep and significant dreams during their vacations, and they brought them into therapy.

Here I must add that in the term vacation I include not only the summer holidays but any occasion during which the individual is removed from his accustomed environment and ordinary preoccupations. One other condition appears requisite: the vacation should not be agitated and exciting; it should rather afford the vacationer a goodly measure of tranquility.

Vacation dreams are singular in that they uncover so much that proves of importance to the patient—as well as, I might add, to me. The more significant result is the immediacy of the insight the patient gains.[8] While the vacation dream is intense, deep, and revealing, it does not effect a cure. It does confront the patient with the challenge innate in the disorder, and thus in a measure points the way to recovery.

It was thinking about the vacation dream that led me to recognize how much it had in common with the incubation dream of the later period of the Asclepian cult. The dynamics of both appear to be clear and parallel.

We dream daily. Ordinarily we recall but few dreams, for we are not attentive, and generally our dreams are bland. But when we are troubled by frustration, adversity, and anxiety we dream intensely, are more aware of our dreams, and can remember and recall them more readily. In the busyness of our everyday life, unless our spirit is taxed and our psyche is under stress, our dreams are freighted and overlaid by, and hence revolve about, our immediate concerns. Though such dreams, as all our dreams, are conditioned by our past, the past in them is submerged.

The deep past is not patent in the commonplace dream, but it *is* in the incubation dream and in the vacation dream. To begin with, both are dreamt under singular circumstances. In both the individual is in retreat, withdrawn, by compelling intention in the case of the patient in the Asclepian Temple, and more freely in the instance of the psychiatric patient on vacation. In these singular circumstances, the individual can better and more clearly hear the voice of his inner self, his unconscious, and this voice can point the way to his psychological and physical salvation.

Aristides, in his *Sacred Orations—Eulogy to Asclepius,* wrote:

> Once I heard the following opinion given as to divine converse and
> intercourse. He said that the mind must be removed from actual
> circumstances, and if that were done, it could consort with the gods,
> and by intercourse would soar above the human state. In this there
> is nothing marvelous, neither the fact that superiority produces inter-
> course with the god, nor that intercourse produces superiority.

The Asclepian temples encouraged and facilitated retreat from
the mundane. Situated, as they commonly were, in setting both pleasant and inspiring, at times magnificent (even today one cannot but
be moved by the grandeur of the temple sites at Cos, Epidaurus, and
Pergamus), ministered by priests, buttressed by the awe-inspiring
presence of the god-spirit—how could the supplicant, the patient, not
shed the trivia of his common life and turn inward to his deeper self.

The Asclepian rites were chthonian in character, and as Edelstein
points out, "The healings themselves were understood by the patients
as revivals; they were reborn through Asclepius."[8] The god spoke
to the ailing supplicant in the incubation dream, giving him counsel
and guidance, pointing when possible (for Asclepius did not pretend
to be omnipotent) the way to recovery.

But then, did he really? Is that which comes down to us in the
ancient records and reports mere fancy, or did Asclepius in effect give
counsel and guidance and lead the sick back to health? We do, of
course, have the testimonies, the recitations, avowals, the votive offer-
ings of those who reported themselves cured by the intercession and
counsel of Asclepius. Edelstein makes much of these testimonies and
grants them high credence. And so would I. But there is even stronger,
more impressive, and more immediate evidence to support the authenticity of what is reported of the Asclepian incubation dream.

We of today may have forgotten Asclepius, or perhaps we are
mindful of him in a different guise and under a different name, but
we have not forgotten how to dream. Among the dreams we dream
are some as deep, as revealing, and proffering the same order of
chthonic insight as did the Asclepian incubation dream. The setting
wherein the dream is dreamt differs, but the dynamics of the vacation
dream are not different from those that evoked the incubation dream:
an earnest and intensive longing for recovery and health, retreat from
the trivia of everyday busyness, a turning inward of the mind's eye
and of the spirit's ear, a readiness to attend to what the inner self
may present, and a willingness as well as a refined competence to
understand—all of which, I believe, calls for sacrifices and purification.

I would like to offer some testimonies, some dreams I have encountered, that could as well have come from the testimonies of
Epidaurus, Cos, or Pergamus.

B.T. was the ugly duckling daughter of a pretty and flirtatious mother who overshadowed her daughter and blighted her youth. In the intense, deep and revealing vacation dream that pointed out the way to recovery, she was eating chicken salad with her mother. Suddenly, looking down on her plate, she perceived that it was her own brain she was eating. The symbolism of that dream brought to the daughter's sudden awareness her helpless, self-destructive relationship to her mother, a prosaic, ambitious, status-seeking parent. Suddenly, she realized that, although mentally superior to the other and animated by higher standards of human behavior, she had succumbed to her manipulating her toward a degrading marriage and, in effect, overpowering her attempts to resist and making her become the consumer of her own autonomy and abilities. This eloquent dream brought about the revival of her authenticity.

T.P. is 28 years of age, in lifelong enmity with his father, but given solace by his mother. He dreams a dream as Sophocles might have conceived it. He is copulating with his sister. His mother appears. He attempts to hide, but is unsuccessful. The mother is aware of everything, frowns disapprovingly and leaves silently. The Sophoclean touch is this! The patient hasn't, and never had, a sister. But in his bondage to the mother, every woman is as a sister to him and taboo. In this dream, the fear has to be faced and the taboo loses its prohibitive rigor. The mother is seen simply frowning, not protesting, and only the event of this vacation dream liberated T.P.

The dream of Miss L. is of the same order but more stark. Miss L. is an attractive and very bright young woman, twenty-three years of age. Her meteoric history includes college matriculation at sixteen, marriage at seventeen, divorce at nineteen, and since then, a painful and seemingly hopeless involvement with a man fifteen years her senior. She will neither wed him, nor separate from him. Why? was her gnawing question. Why? Then, she dreamt this dream, cited verbatim.[9] John is with her, and it is thus she tells of her dream:

> Suddenly he was facing me, [that is, John] very close, and saying "But don't you think I have taken over those functions of your father, become like a father substitute?" These words echo like needles [sic] into me. He kind of has the quality of screaming in his voice. He is saying something like K's mother [the mother of her divorced husband] said about my meeting K so early at college, making it easier for me to adjust to the situation with my family. I keep denying. He thinks this is something good, but I know, somehow, that it is horrible, and I am ashamed. . . .
>
> We are again in an apartment, in the living room, having an awful fight. He is yelling at me ferociously. I run into the bathroom hysterically and lock the door—I think I am trying to brush my teeth. I am crying and he is pounding on the door. Suddenly he breaks the

door down, and it is not John. It is my father, naked, and he is saying he will kill me if I don't do something. I am screaming and he
is about to hit me with his body when I wake up.

Asclepius could afford her no clearer insight, nor point more
sharply the way to her salvation. Miss L.'s vacation dream is significant in its resemblance to the incubation dream, that is, it is remarkable for the completeness with which it uncovers the repressed
knowledge in one single oneiric experience. The dream tells not only
the meaning of each of Miss L.'s three significant sexual attachments
but why she could so successfully repress her problem and why her
attempt to act it out with a substitute was unsuccessful. John, the substitute figure, speaks for himself but in the dream, he also unmasks
the young former husband's role as a partner to a previous attempt
to solve her problem concerning the father, that is, a vain effort to
escape him. It finally tells why she, a brilliant young woman of this
era, could be so baffled about her obvious problem and even could not
resolve it after it hit her squarely with overwhelming immediacy but
simultaneously with a shocking starkness that she could not face.

The following dream was dreamt by P.H., a young woman who,
I am most certain, knew nothing of Asclepius or the dreams of Aristagora or Arata. However, the symbolism of her dream and the ancient
dream we have alluded to are similar. The vernacular of P.H.'s dream
is modern, the motif as old as civilization, but the incubation dream
can articulate in its ancient tongue, even today. I cite this dream of
P.H. from my records, somewhat abridged.

> We are planning to get married. Last day for working there and I
> do something wrong or something happens. Anyway, I am to be
> beheaded. At first, don't really take it seriously. Gradually, I realize
> that I am really going to be beheaded. Start trying to think of ways to
> get out of it. The execution is going to take place on a special boat on
> the river. Somehow gets to be a whole group of girls that is going to
> be beheaded. Something about girls simply not being able to handle
> something on board ship correctly and therefore have to die. Nobody
> is being very wholehearted about executions, but has to go ahead.
> I am still terribly ambivalent whether to try and escape or not. There
> is some concept that we will revive, but be rather lifeless or some-
> how changed. In the meantime, the first girl is being made to hold
> her neck over a pot of boiling water in preparation for the knife and
> I begin to realize the full impact of what is happening. Some fellow
> outside the door stands guard, but he is cooperating with my running
> away. Calls boy friend, who is out hunting, and tells him to go back
> to the ship with the bloody knife to cover up my running away.

The interpretation of this dream is simple enough. It is an anxiety dream in which the dreamer wrestles with the problem of pre-marital intercourse and the fear of defloration. The phallic significance of the knife is patent; the play on the menace of "going to be be-headed" (the loss of the maidenhead) is Freudian to the nth degree. The noteworthy feature of this dream, as in the dreams of Aristagora and Arata, is this: The severed head is to be restituted. "We will re-vive," the dreamer affirms. Clearly then, the issues may differ, but the vernacular is the same in the incubation as in the vacation dream. We forego entering into the additional revelatory aspects of this dream. We are built on the same archetype. Whatever the number of variations we compose, the basic theme is archaic and common to mankind.

Here end "my testimonies." Here also ends a minor exposition on what I would title "The Utility of Medicine in Medical History." Medical experience and thought of today provide the clues for a deeper understanding of past periods and the verification of their claims of help and cure to the sick. The utility of the physician who aimed primarily at cure and alleviation of "ills," however, transcends their circumscribed task. To become a healing agent, the physician must understand man in his being and becoming, in the climate of his time, and within the institutions he creates, maintains, and dis-cards. This essay is intended as a verification through modern knowl-edge, experience, and insight of the meaning and utility of ancient methods of cure. The similarity of the symbolism of the ancient and modern troubled dreamer is a gauge for the similarity of the process of cure and, therefore, a validation. Medical history has demonstrated here the utility of medicine, one of man's institutions that has endured.

References

1. Hamilton, Mary, *Incubation or The Cure of Disease in Pagan Temples and Christian Churches* (London: Simkin, Marshall, Hamilton, Kent Co., 1906), p. 2.
2. Edelstein, Emma J. and Ludwig, *Asclepius: A Collection and Inter-pretation of The Testimonies* (Baltimore: Johns Hopkins Press, 1945), vol. I, p. 235, test. 33.
3. Ibid., vol. I, p. 32, test. 12.
4. Ibid., vol. I, pp. 229–237.
5. Hamilton, Mary, op. cit. (in reference 1), p. 70.
6. Ibid., p. 42.
7. Edelstein, op. cit. (in reference 2), vol. II, p. 173.
8. Ibid.
9. Galdston, Iago, "An Existential Analysis of the Case of Miss. L." in *Existential Analysis*, (Chicago: 1963).

R. Volmat and F. Dufay

7

"De Planetarum Influxu": The Artistic Production of a Chronic Untreated Delirious Subject

The archaic, unfathomable forces of destruction have preoccupied man's mind whether they strike from outside in nature as incomprehensible destiny or spring from dark sources within and between men. Myth and legend are witnesses to this effect. Greek tragedy viewed man as the victim of an inexorable destiny, although conflict was foreshadowed in the tragedies of the later period. The pangs of conflict appear more clearly in the great tragedies of the sixteenth and seventeenth centuries. Only since the archaic or the unconscious manifestations in man have entered the observational field of the psychological sciences has their destructive impact been discovered to be inside man. More and more clearly has the unconscious or irrational mind emanated as an antagonist to the advances of the human rational mind and as deficient in the idiom by which to communicate with its enlightened but frail ruler, the rational mind. Increasingly, that flexible instrument searched for communication with its archaic precursor, thus aiming at control over it. As the master of the unconscious antagonist, the rational mind builds a world and societies of its own, and anticipates the future.

Man has made progress towards the goal of communication in interpreting body language and hidden meaning underlying human behavior, in particular, artistic expression. Understandably, the sick became a primary object of observation and source of an ever-enriched pool of comprehension. In Freudian terms, the sublimated artistic forms of expression are the manifestations of repressed unconscious forces. In the evolutionary neuropsychiatric view, such achievements must be considered as the surviving functions unleashed by the defective control of these higher levels of functioning. It shows the sick person in his reduced state of integration,[1] a factor that the following case confirms, even when in accordance with Freud we consider the patient's art work as sublimation. Sublimation should be considered a self-healing tendency, as the case presented below will demonstrate.

Our subject is a fifty-four-year-old man, who, despite a delirious mental illness of twenty years' duration, has never been the subject of a psychiatric consultation. We have attempted from the case history and from the artistic work itself, to discover the principal personality traits of this man.

He was born in 1920, in a village where nothing ever happened that would have prompted him to leave. A bachelor, he lives with his mother on the family farm, which his two older sisters abandoned for marriage and from which his father left for the village cemetery in 1948.

A door, which he opens to persons whom he considers learned, leads into a passageway where rest his latest creations, which have not been disregarded by either the local press or television. At the end of the passageway is the "Museum," where the patient hoards the works executed between 1955 and 1965; the door of the museum room symbolizes the drying up of creativity in 1965, following a spinal injury when the patient was a porter.

Our patient is a stocky man, given to chameleon-like mimicry, with piercing eyes expressing disproportionate emotions: A jovial expression can be suddenly cut off, to be replaced by a look of interrogation that scrutinizes the physiognomy of his interlocutor for total adherence. The output of his discourse is rapid; he instills, or force-feeds, us with words. He is aided by that unconditional priestess which his mother has become. This verbal affluence appears to be polyvalent. Its character of release may be supported by the anxiety attendant to the lack of control, by a fear of drain and a resultant void. On the one hand, the profuseness of this verbal flow serves his proselytism, the spread of his messianic frenzy, his cosmic and mystic ecstasy. He crowds his ideas of grandeur with realistic assertions in the attempt to make his pronouncements more assimilable by the simultaneous negation of his uncovered irrationality. In resorting to this foothold on reality, he reveals a self-healing tendency that also keeps open the channels of communication with his learned audience.

Three stages are distinguishable in our subject's choice of his artistic medium. They obviously correspond to the message emanating from his inner experiences. We seem justified in assuming in this process a development reflected in the interaction with the material as well as with his artistic projections.

THE EVALUATION OF THE ARTISTIC MEDIUM

After having traced a map [of the two surfaces of Mars], the subject has the idea in 1955 of using quick-setting cement in a pure state to materialize what has swarmed in his mind since the death of his father and to bring a little order to his imagination, nourished with audioverbal and visual hallucinations. He first produces two-dimensional pictures, attacking the problem in the yielding mass, which in hardening fast will unalterably obey his will. He proceeds to the construction of modeled statues in mixed mortar, representing objects or people, earthly or otherwise. In 1972, emerging from a period of posttraumatic despondency, he again takes up artistic production; abandoning the modeling that permitted him to construct a world from mortar, he attacks sculpture, in which he must pit himself against solid mineral masses.

The meaningful correspondence between the material chosen and the depicted feelings or visions reveals the stages of adjustment made by the patient to his world. Having overcome dream, hope, and desire, a period of attempted reality adjustment, the terror of the one exposed to the deluding world, he finally harmonizes his tamed self with a subjugated environment. Actually, we are confronted with the patient's autobiography expressed pictorially and by the medium of sculpture. These pictures combine elements that correspond to the artistic projections of the mentally ill: the emotional impact of the self-symbolized by the tree, the theme of the obstacle, the unsafe water and land expressing ambivalence, the bestiary, while monsters will, little by little, complete the panoply.

THE EVOLUTION OF THE ARTISTIC MEDIUM AND SYMBOLISM OF THE ARTISTIC PRODUCT

The earliest productions are picturesque; they represent negatives of the bas-relief idea. They do not radiate at first sight a disquieting strangeness. We see a woman in an attractive landscape shielding in her arms a half-kneeling lamb to whom flock three other sheep by order of size. The youngest, at the greatest distance, steps down from an elevated, meadowy knoll. At further scrutiny, this picture already announces a conflictual situation, reflecting a dawning disclosure within the patient's mind of a premonitory awareness that will emanate more clearly as his work unfolds before us. The mothering woman is a little Jeanne d'Arc with harsh, masculine traits; but more ominous seems the bird perched off to one side. Its desperately open beak already symbolizing menacing rapaciousness begotten by need, we may assume that the picture reveals a long-standing yearning. His conjuring on the picture could neither fulfill this dream nor appease the ensuing rising frustration.

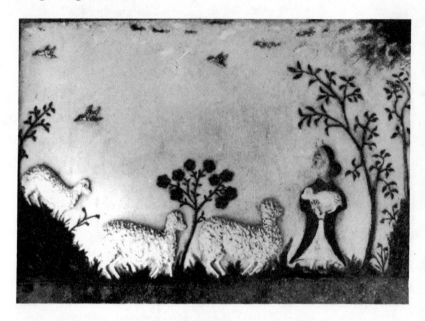

The next picture is more explicit of avidity for nurture. A lonely fawn stands with his hind legs on arid, craggy, and steep terrain, his whole body stretched out toward a branch of leaves overhead. The landscape and the posture of the fawn depict the contrast of his isolated stand on sterile ground and the unattainable distance to the promising leaves nearby. The painful deprivation of the animal, with his useless forefeet and only the oral area with stretched out tongue as an organ to reach for the leaves, is impressively disclosed. The effort of the whole body of this being in a desolate surrounding that beckons and simultaneously denies evokes the atmosphere of Tantalus in the Greek hell. There is the difference that this truly dramatic creature is still, as in the former picture, the symbol of an unoffensive animal, a symbol of artless exposure to false lure and vain effort. The first sign of danger can be gathered from the precarious balance in which the pathetic animal finds itself searching for the nearest leaf on a branch that covers the length of the top of the picture. Losing balance would expose him infallibly to being pierced by two bifurcated branches protruding toward his back. This picture was actually the patient's first creation; he had discarded it in a shameful endeavor to hide it. Game appears in another of his pictures, which illustrates a couple under the scrutinizing eye of a predator in a deadly atmosphere.

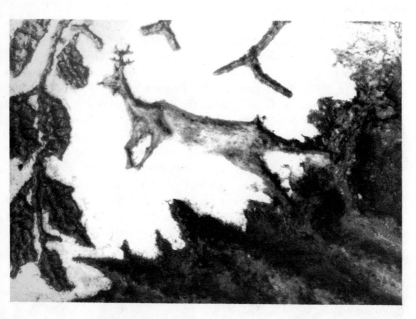

We are inclined to see in these artistic productions a gigantic effort of the sick to cope with an alluring but deceptive world and thereby with himself. Symbolization of the artless, innocent, peaceful, and exposed animal is evident in the three bas-relief models in cement. One could call the first two pictures allegories, the deceptive security and the deceptive promise of nurture. If we see in the hungry, open-beaked bird on the tree menacing the lamb the first unsheltering omen of threatening destruction, the awareness of a menacing rapaciousness begotten by need, we are on the trail of a confusion of identity, the gentle and menaced, and the rapacious and destructive self in a similar antithetic world that, therefore, deserves cautious scrutiny.

The transitory phase from two dimensional to three dimensional art is not made without paying tribute to nature: a lily, an orange tree that the patient prizes highly and that is coveted by children, and a barge loaded with flowers.

The first sculpture in mortar retains the identification with a symbol of gentleness, the dove. The bird sits as if impaled upon an aggressively thorny stalk, which, in his interpretation, proves to be the umbilical cord. Fidelity to the color white persists, confirmed by the symbolic values of the lily and the dove. Most revealing is a form that represents a heart with the ambivalent coloring of black at its apex as well as its base, and white walled in between the blackness. Its identity with the womb, the desired object of begetting love, becomes clear in the artist-patient's explanation that this thorny stalk is the umbilical cord on which is impaled the dove, another symbol of his longing for gentle and peaceful identity, aggressively attacked and held captured. Aspects of flag-waving reveal themselves at the level of the heart, upholding the dove. This patriotic enthusiasm reaches a climax in the armless bust of the brigadier general, who is none other than General de Gaulle. He is the only unmistakably male figure and the patient's presumable ideal image conjured into mortar. It appears as a turning point in the patient's development, a move from the unoffensive creature dependent on care and gratification to identification with a male person representing strength and glory. However, he has not reached the freedom of ideal formation and has to rely on the creation of a tangible portrait for the permanence and solidity of his identification. The still-inoffensive, friendly expression of the sculptured physiognomy is aloof and devoid of any vitality and promise. The glance is introverted, yet scrutinizing. The valorous effort again fails.

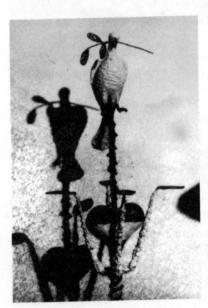 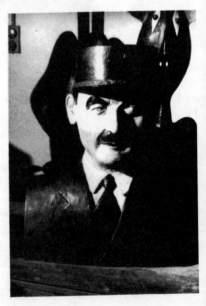

The return to the symbiotic "thorny" relation to the mother is inescapable. The ambivalence of the relation is now depicted more realistically in a bipolar portrait of two women sculpted in mortar.

Its chronologic place following the only sculptured likeness of a realistic human male is strongly suggestive of the meaning these sculptures express. It is as though despite the degree of permanence conveyed to the solidified mortar, self-sufficiency cannot be realized. Resort to female support follows, but her identity as a natural mother is denied. She is a virgin, double featured, remodeled in the same black and white contrast as the deceptive heart-womb, symbolically emitting the thorny umbilical cord, and thus impaling the dove. He interprets the differences between the two virgins in form and colors whose oneness is expressed by their finding a womb in an available gilded vase. He explains that the white virgin is associated with human beings, the black virgin is otherworldly; she is the patient's springboard when he plunges into delirious alienation escaping an overpowering reality.

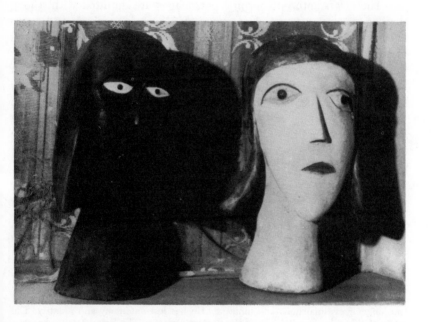

As if to avoid any torment resulting from desires and fears he undergoes when he is fully awake, he lets his mind drift. The subject first hallucinates, then reproduces physically asexual beings that do not belong to our world, live most of the time in swamps, draw up the juice of the planet through suckers, but are provided with filters that protect them against poisoning. The earth becomes the nurturing mother, but contrary to Thomas Mann's Holy Sinner, not purifying, not making one the elected. One's effort of filtering its poison is not delivering. More and more the patient is overwhelmed by what he fears, fights, and abhors. He cannot achieve self-identification. The more he struggles, the more the limits are effaced between himself and the dangerous mother who has become ubiquitous, the whole world.

The personages created by the patient are not attractive, but the horror that they arouse comes more from the intentions and sentiments projected by their creator than from their physical aspect, whether or not it is anthropomorphic.

The most "human" personage possesses arms and legs, but his upper extremities make of him a robot in the pay of sadistic Martians who surround him. They will take "human samples" thanks to the little pincers of this artificial demon, who moves about easily through the swamps because he has feet like little barges. A diabolic arsenal is completed by eyes capable of darting paralyzing, if not lethal, rays.°

These less-anthropomorphic personages are outfitted with a long slender tail and a crown of antennae divided into receivers and transmitters, and display a characteristic want of upper limbs as this god of another planet. He springs from a floral receptacle and weeps over the events reported to him by two of the three horns that serve him as antennae, while the third permits him to distribute advice that is never listened to. The extremities of other figures are most often webbed, in keeping with an unstable terrain; each is provided with antennae with multiple ends about which the patient knows all the secrets, his mission being to warn human beings of what is being plotted against them.

°In reference to the autobiographical development revealed by these artistic manifestations, the following comment might be in order. The two Martians on each side are abstract symbols of complementary sexuality; the female symbol again is duplicated. The robot squeezed in between but slightly in front of the figures stretches his stiff, inarticulate arms, each ending in a dart, to both sides symbolizing stymieing ambivalence. The robot impresses one as a sexually neutralized, inescapably subjugated automat wound up for the restricted action to which he is designed by the unscrutable, dehumanized abstract powers. The patient no longer feels innocuous and innocent. He has lost autonomy and identity. The eyes of this robot remind one of the patient's glance. The hare-like ears bespeak alertness to the deceptiveness of the world and fear of involvement with rapaciousness for which the robot's open mouth, with its canine teeth, is well equipped. We shall witness the further process of self-alienation, not without morbid, futile, superhuman attempts of finding communication at cosmic or archaeological distances, in the resources of the animal realm with the surroundings. This latter adaptation reminds one of archaic man's borrowing strength and skills from the heads and hides of feared and admired animals. This patient, however, attempts adaptation in a more versatile way. His sweep over the animal resources is broader. His creatures have webbed feet to move with security over the everlasting marshy insecurity of the earthly world. They have receptive and emiting antennae and clutch-like claws and wings.

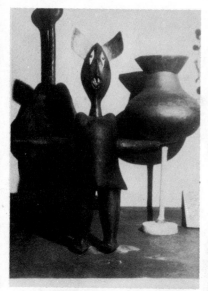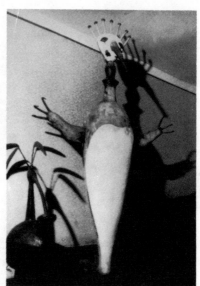

Zoomorphic characteristics are distributed among an animal of antediluvian aspect with threatening jaws, magnetic eyes, and greedy nostrils; a sort of giraffe possessing, besides usual equipment, a grating for a mouth; and several avian monsters with beaks and webbed feet, among whom a penguin with hooks represents a dangerous specimen. The glutted serpent, a great boa that charms its victims before crunching their flesh in its infernal jaws, digests slowly in an almost "injaculatory" peristalsis the blood that colors its skin; a monster standing on four slender paws is described to us as hiding in clumps of sea flowers in order to suck sadistically the blood of the victims he terrifies, his eyes bloodshot with the sap of his prey. Finally, an inoffensive being raises his eyes to heaven to implore a gift that his antennae are seeking on the ground.

The color red, which is found again and again, appears on the body and in bloodshot eyes, which is an ill omen since, in the opinion of one of the authors, "negatively, red is the symbol of war, of destruction." Black also is represented in contrast with red or blended with the green of the camouflage service dress.

So we find ourselves confronted with monstrous beings equipped to survive in an unstable and barren milieu, where sex is not in its place but aggressiveness is widely supplied, and where each organ, by its presence or absence, can represent the sexual function at its different stages when one refers to oneiric symbolism.

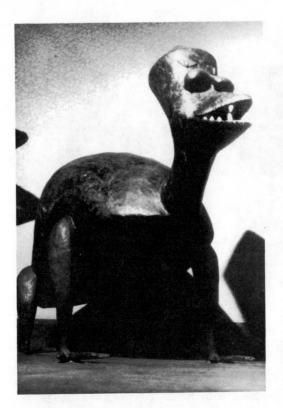
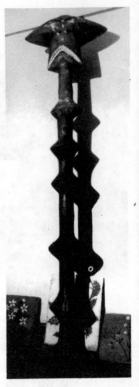

The art of bas-relief practiced for two years by the patient has enabled him to imprint in stone bodies in which sex is suggested through the medium of breasts, appearing in aggressive relief in the little dancer; this figure, one of three feminine bas-relief statues is devoid of upper extremities, as if the notion of arms, in its intimate phallic repercussions, were intolerable to the patient; the theme of water is found again in the mermaid. These subjects, whether a human head or carvings deriving from bird or fish, run no risk of being harmful, concealed as they are in their eternity.

Upon entering the museum we take a leap into a world peopled with malevolent intentions, with unpunished extortions, created by the patient, who establishes himself as the arbiter of the persecutory and unwholesome activities of his creations and of the surrounding world.

At the juncture of these two worlds, the hinge of a gigantic primitive scene, he exercises his full powers, practicing the art of projection by identification with the beings that he "procreates." The capacity and device of symbolic projection liberates him from the urge to

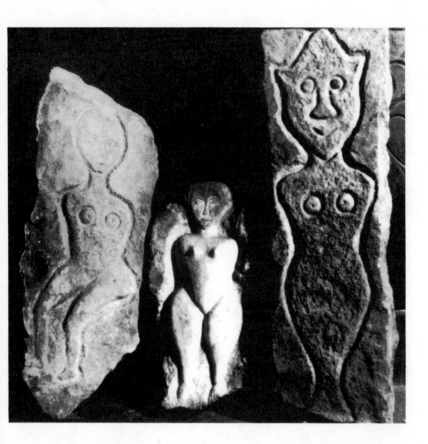

attribute to beings other than the creatures of his fantasies qualities, sentiments, and desires that he fails to recognize or repudiates in himself. It heals him from retaliating against any other person than the images of his projected feelings or qualities.

His Titanic labors in the world of preserved people and the world populated by his creativeness—where the needy becomes the menace and the menace expresses need—in rendering him less alone have satisfied the narcissism of our delirious subject if, with Freud, we admit that "the individual feels incomplete when he is alone."

REFERENCE

1. Walther Riese, "The Principle of Integration, Its History and Its Nature," *Journal of Nervous and Mental Disease*, 96:296–312, 1942.

Part III

Medical Historians
Study Their Masters
and Great Men of the Past

In this section, Thomas Jefferson, Heinrich Heine, and three great physicians—Zimmermann, Cabanis, and Jung—are studied against the background of their periods and personal origins. Jarcho discusses a group of scientists who contributed by their self-observation to the discovery and minute description of the optic phenomena in migraine. In particular, through self-observation Wollaston confirmed Newton's assumption that the optic nerve was semidecussated (i.e., not completely crossing to the opposite side of the brain; consequently, an affect to the nerve may produce only unilateral symptoms). To the creative introversion of the astronomers and natural philosophers studied in this section, we owe findings we expect from the physician. The questions arise whether this phenomenon is due to the physician's being distracted by extroversive aspects of his profession, whether it partly explains why a dichotomy has developed between the practicing physician or specialist and the researcher who withdraws to his laboratory, and whether the collective and team aspects of modern research will cause the researcher also to become distracted by merely prolific performance and, in turn, lose his creative introversion.

Veith explores solitude and loneliness and interprets them as "stages of mind" rather than symptoms of isolation and alienation. She rejects the notion of solitude as a means of self-search or withdrawal from worldliness to become close to the divine. Her examples of those pursuing solitude for self-search are Montaigne in his study and Rousseau amidst nature, whereas manifestations of withdrawal from worldliness are such historical movements as hermitism in both Eastern and Western religions. Veith raises the question whether the attractiveness of Greta Garbo, the modern film actress, was of a mystical nature or a nostalgia felt by the gregarious American people for their former need of privacy. Solitude was considered contrary to the essence of woman. To the religiously withdrawn, she was the image of earthly impurity. Even female animals were excluded from the Coptic monasteries, which were built on nearly inaccessible mountaintops. Similar searches for purity were pursued in Japanese Zen monasteries. Unlike today, married monks had to leave wives, families, and all worldly connections. Veith quotes a reflection by Terence on man's self-love, and appears to brush away with a smile men's obliviousness of their dependence on woman. They forget that Adam would still be alone in paradise, were it not for Eve's existence, and that he would still be with an immaculate Eve, were it not for her curiosity. To this curiosity the monks owe their remote birth and aspiration toward God in the company of others who are also her heirs.

The major portion of Veith's study is devoted to the life and work of the Swiss physician Johann Zimmerman. For his creativity he needed solitude, but it conflicted with his social tendencies. He was a contemporary of Lessing, and the elegiac mood of his life and the subjectivity of its preoccupations foreshadowed German Romanticism.

By contrast, Heine lived and wrote in the Romantic period without being a "child of his period." Schachter discusses Heine's personality and disease. About both, Schachter deplores the insufficient data, which prevent full clarification. However, he emphasizes two of Heine's traits, which also belonged to two of his male ancestors: riotous living in youth and indifference in dealing with money. Schachter questions whether these traits were not due to Heine's sensitive reaction to being slighted as a Jew, for he had been slighted despite his academic and creative merits and despite his self-betrayal, the religious conversion necessary before society would recognize his merits. His emotional condition and its psychosomatic manifestations stood in the way of a discernment of these symptoms from the ones produced by the organic disease, and, therefore, prevented a clarification of the differential diagnosis. The religious conversion troubled him throughout his life, and in his last years, he made a confession of Jewish faith. In addition to the Old Testament—the "portable fatherland of the Jews," as he called it—he carried the baggage of Western humanistic civilization without ever establishing any true earthly roots. This rootlessness had been the Jewish destiny for two millennia.

The opposite impression is produced by Ellenberger's study of Carl Jung. Through the historical setting of three generations, Ellenberger traces the multiple factors that shaped Jung's theories—in particular, the theory of individuation. An intricate network of internal gropings and family interaction is traced, and different aspects of Jung's family background are compared. Current versions of that background are based on family traditions and stories, but documentary evidence suggests an "unknown history" consisting of facts that the family distorted, concealed, or forgot. The multigenerational focus of the article evokes Jung's aphorism that "nothing is more important in the destiny of a man than the life his parents have not lived." This aphorism implies that, to be himself, Jung had actively to free himself from his unconscious familial ties and join the etymological filaments that unite all mankind in "collective" ties of communication.

Whereas Heine was frustrated in his search for universal human affiliation and Jung found the ties of universal communication in the unconscious, Jefferson, Cabanis, and the circle of the ideologues discussed by Mora were united by the spirit of the age of enlightened rationality. The mission these men fulfilled for mankind seems to transcend their time and so dwarf the setting in which their inspirational thought and action occurred. Yet the setting was important. The germ of their thinking had been planted in England by Locke and in France by Condillac. When Franklin introduced Jefferson to the group of ideologues who gathered in the home of the inspiring Madame Helvétius, Jefferson did not come unprepared. He was already part of the community of the scientific and humanitarian spirit and had already begun to set into motion his concerns for legislation to protect the unsound of mind. Cabanis was keenly interested in the same problem, but he was more of a theoretician than Jefferson, who remained throughout his life a man of action. Nevertheless, it is due to Cabanis that action was instituted in France. He recommended Pinel to the post of head physician at the Bicêtra Hospital, and there Pinel could implement the human rights of the mentally ill and inspire generations of physicians and thinkers who increasingly recognized and served their needs.

Reading Mora, we become aware of how lasting this impulse has been and how slow the progress. Our generation is struggling to improve the still inadequate treatment of the mentally ill. We are still handicapped by our ways of imprisoning them, be it in hospitals or in the straitjacket of psychotropic drugs that merely subdue them. But the humanitarian conscience spread by the rationalistic elite of the past is alive today in democratic countries, and their citizens enjoy a wider spirit of alertness. In addition, science has begun to understand the irrational in man and particularly in the mentally ill. Yet it is in the inspired leaders of the past that such enlightenment and progress originated. Mora's essay discusses each of these luminous minds, their mutual relationship, and the specific contribution their dedication has made to the cause of humanitarianism and the spirit of science. It is uplifting to perceive both the aid they gave unselfishly to each other and the faith that caused them to send their findings across the ocean to touch kindred minds on foreign shores.

Saul Jarcho

8

Self-Observation by Astronomers and "Natural Philosophers"

In Charles Hilton Fagge's *Principles and Practice of Medicine*,[1] one of the best medical textbooks ever written, the following remarkable statement occurs in the section on migraine:

> A very curious circumstance in regard to the visual affection is that some of the best and most careful descriptions of it have been written, not by medical men, but by astronomers and natural philosophers. Wollaston, Arago, Sir David Brewster, Sir John Herschel, Sir Charles Wheatstone, Du Bois Reymond, Sir George Airy, and Professor Dufour, of Lausanne, may be mentioned as having been liable to this paroxysmal defect of sight, and as having carefully noted its phenomena; and no similar malady has, within the present century, been the subject of two papers admitted into the "Philosophical Transactions," as well as of communications to the "Philosophical Magazine" and other scientific journals at home and abroad. It may be a question whether persons who are not accustomed to employ the eyes for minute observation would notice the dimness of sight, or regard it as of sufficient importance to be mentioned to their physician. Indeed, when it commences at some distance from the centre of vision, I believe it is sure to be overlooked, unless the patient's attention is specially directed to its occurrence. And this may, perhaps, be the reason why Professor Du Bois Reymond does not mention it in describing this form of headache as he has experienced it himself.

A search for the scientists and the descriptions mentioned by Fagge revealed a plenitude of interesting material.[2] The first author

---

Reprinted with permission from the *Bulletin of the New York Academy of Medicine*, 4:886, 1968 (original title: "Migraine in Astronomers and 'Natural Philosophers'").

in point of time is William Hyde Wollaston (1766–1828), M.B. 1788, M.D. 1793, the gifted physicist and chemist who discovered palladium and rhodium, invented a method for welding pure platinum, created numerous optical devices, and contributed an early study of the solar spectrum.[3] Since 1800 Wollaston had had occasional attacks of bilateral partial blindness. In 1824 further observation of his hemianopsia led him to the opinion—previously advanced by Sir Isaac Newton[4]—that the optic nerves were semidecussated. Wollaston reported his observations as follows:[5]

> It is now more than twenty years since I was first affected with the peculiar state of vision, to which I allude, in consequence of violent exercise I had taken for two or three hours before. I suddenly found that I could see but half the face of a man whom I met; and it was the same with respect to every object I looked at. In attempting to read the name JOHNSON, over a door, I saw only   SON; the commencement of the name being wholly obliterated to my view. In this instance the loss of sight was toward my left, and was the same whether I looked with the right eye or the left. This blindness was not so complete as to amount to absolute blackness, but was a shaded darkness without definite outline. The complaint was of short duration, and in about a quarter of an hour might be said to be wholly gone, having receded with a gradual motion from the center of vision obliquely upwards toward the left.
>
> Since this defect arose from over fatigue, a cause common to many other nervous affections, I saw no reason to apprehend any return of it, and it passed away without my drawing any useful inference from it.
>
> It is now about fifteen months since a similar affection occurred again to myself, without my being able to assign any cause whatever, or to connect it with any previous or subsequent indisposition. The blindness was first observed, as before, in looking at the face of a person I met, whose *left* eye was to my sight obliterated. My blindness was in this instance the reverse of the former, being to *my right* (instead of the left) of the spot to which my eyes were directed; so that I have no reason to suppose it in any manner connected with the former affection.

It is of additional interest that Wollaston died in 1828 of brain tumor.

In 1824 François Arago (1786–1853), the astronomer and physicist, published a French translation of Wollaston's paper.[6] To this he subjoined an editorial note[7] in which he stated:

> The affection described by M. Wollaston, is quite common. I know four persons who are subject to it, and I myself have had three attacks in the last month. The first and second times I could not see things

situated to the right of the axis of vision. The third time, on September 27, 1824, objects on the right were, on the contrary, the only ones I could see. For example, having directed my gaze at the right limb of the M of the word BAROMETRE, which was written in large characters above an instrument, I could see this stroke perfectly and also the remaining letters ETRE, but I could not see at all either the first upstroke of the M or the BARO. Whichever eye I used, the same phenomenon prevailed. A headache appeared on the right side above the eye twenty minutes later when the half-blindness ceased. . . .

On February 20, 1865, Sir David Brewster (1781–1868), the famous physicist, eminent for studies of optical phenomena, read before the Royal Society of Edinburgh a paper titled *On Hemiopsy, or Half-Vision.*[8] Brewster wrote:

. . . Having myself experienced several attacks of hemiopsy, I have been enabled to ascertain the optical condition of the retina when under its influence, and to determine the extent of the affection, and its immediate cause.

In reading the different cases of hemiopsy, we are led to infer that there is vision in one-half of the retina, and blindness in the other. But this is not the case. The blindness, or insensibility to distinct impressions, exists chiefly in a small portion of the retina to the right or left hand of the *foramen centrale,* and extends itself irregularly to other parts of the retina on the same side, in the neighborhood of which the vision is uninjured. In some cases the upper half of the object is invisible, the part of the retina paralyzed being a little below the *foramen centrale.* On some occasions, in absolute darkness, when a faint glow of light was produced by some uniform pressure upon the whole of the retina, I have observed a great number of black spots, corresponding to parts of the retina upon which no pressure was exerted.

In the case of ordinary hemiopsy, as observed by myself, there is neither darkness nor obscurity, the portion of the paper from which the letters disappear being as bright as those upon which they are seen. Now, this is a remarkable condition of the retina. While it is sensible to luminous impressions, it is insensible to the lines and shades of the pictures which it receives of external objects; or, in other words, the retina is in certain parts of it in such a state that the light which falls upon it is irradiated, or passes into the dark lines or shades of the pictures upon it, and obliterates them.

The most valuable of the older descriptions of migraine was composed by Sir George Biddell Airy (1801-92), the Astronomer Royal. Airy wrote as follows:[9]

I have myself been frequently attacked by it, certainly not fewer than twenty times, probably much oftener; and I am acquainted with two persons who have suffered from it, one of them at least a hundred times. From the information of my friends, and from my own experience, I am able to supply an account of some features of the malady which appear to have escaped the notice of Dr. Wollaston and Sir David Brewster. . . .

I discover the beginning of the attack by a little indistinctness in some object at which I am looking directly; and I believe the locality of this indistinctness upon the retina to be, not the place of entrance of the optic nerve, but the centre of the usual field of vision. Very soon I perceive that the indistinctness is caused by the image being crossed by short lines which change their direction and place. In a little time the disease takes its normal type, and presents successively the appearances shown in the following diagram. [See Figure.] In drawing this, I have supposed that the principal obscuration of objects is apparently on the left side; by reversing the figure, left to right, the appearances will be given which present themselves when the principal obscuration appears to be on the right side. (In my own experience, I believe it is an even chance whether the obscuration is to the right or to the left.) The bounding circle shows roughly the extent to which the eye is sensible of vision more or less vivid. Only one arch is seen at one time: The arch is small at first, and gradually increases in dimensions.

The zigzags nearly resemble those in the ornaments of a Norman arch, but are somewhat sharper. Those near the letter B, C, D, E are much deeper than those near b, c, d, e. The zigzags do not change their relative arrangement during the dilatation of the arch, but they tremble strongly: the trembling near B, C, D, E is much greater than that near b, c, d, e. There is a slight appearance of scarlet color on one edge, the external edge, I believe, of the zigzags. As the arch enlarges vision becomes distinct in the centre of the field. The strongly-trembling extremity of the arch rises at the same time that it passes to the left, and finally passes from the visible field, and the whole phenomenon disappears.

I have never been able to decide with certainty whether the disease really affects both eyes. The first impression on the mind is that only one eye is affected (in the instance depicted above, the left eye). There is general obscurity on one side; but the tremor and boiling are so oppressive, that, if produced only in one, they may nearly extinguish the corresponding vision in the other.

The duration of this ocular derangement with me is usually from twenty to thirty minutes, but with one of my friends it sometimes lasts much longer. In general, I feel no further inconvenience from it; but with my friends, it is followed by oppressive headache. . . .

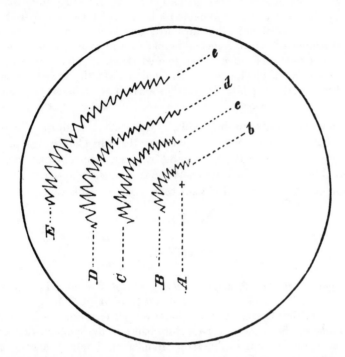

Figure. Disturbance of the visual field in migraine. Drawing by Sir George B. Airy, Astronomer Royal. Reprinted from *London, Edinb., and Dubl. Phil. Mag.*, ser. 4, 30:19–21, 1865. A, the beginning of the disease. Bb, Cc, Dd, Ee, successive appearances, as the arch gradually enlarges.

Those who lay stress on psychic predispositions will read with interest the description of Sir George Airy that appears at the beginning of his autobiography.[10]

> The ruling feature of his [Sir George Airy's] character was undoubtedly Order. From the time that he went up to Cambridge to the end of his life his system of order was strictly maintained. He wrote his autobiography up to date soon after he had taken his degree, and made his first will as soon as he had any money to leave. His accounts were perfectly kept by double entry throughout his life, and he valued extremely the order of book-keeping: this facility of keeping accounts was very useful to him. He seems not to have destroyed a document of any kind whatever: counterfoils of old cheque-books, notes for tradesmen, circulars, bills, and correspondence of all sorts

were carefully preserved in the most complete order from the time
that he went to Cambridge; and a huge mass they formed. To a high
appreciation of order he attributed in a great degree his command
of mathematics, and sometimes spoke of mathematics as nothing more
than a system of order carried to a considerable extent. In everything
he was methodical and orderly, and he had the greatest dread of
disorder creeping into the routine work of the Observatory, even in
the smallest matters.

Elsewhere in his autobiography[11] Airy states that during the meetings of the British Association that were held in Cambridge in June
1833 he had Sir David Brewster and Mr. [John] Herschel as his guests
and breakfasted with them daily. We may wonder whether these three
migrainous astronomers discussed their common affliction.

References

1. Fagge, C. H. *The Principles and Practice of Medicine,* Pye-Smith, P.
   H., ed.; 2d ed. London, Churchill, 1888, vol. 1, p. 781.
2. Emil Du Bois-Reymond, having observed his own cases of hemicrania,
   considered the ailment to be a disturbance of the sympathetic nervous
   system. See his "Zur Kenntniss der Hemikrania," *Arch. f. Anat. Physiol.
   u. Wissensch. Med.,* 1860, pp. 461–68.
3. Hartog, P. J. and Lees, C. H. William Hyde Wollaston. In: *Dictionary
   of National Biography,* vol. 21. London, Oxford Univ. Press, 1921–
   1922, pp. 782–87.
4. Newton, I. *Opticks* (London, 1730). Reprinted from 4th ed. [London,
   1730]. London, Bell, 1931, pp. 346–47.
5. Wollaston, W. H. On Semi-Decussation of the Optic Nerves. *Phil.
   Trans.* 114:222–31, 1824.
6. Wollaston, W. H. De la semi-décussation das nerfs optiques. *Ann. de
   Chimie et de Physique* 27:102–09, 1824.
7. *Ann. de Chimie et de Physique* 27:109–10, 1824.
8. Brewster, D. On Hemiopsy, or Half-Vision, *London, Edinb., and Dublin
   Phil. Mag.,* ser. 4, 29:503–07, 1865. Reprinted in *Trans. Roy. Soc.
   Edinb.* 24:15–18, 1867.
9. Airy, G. B. The Astronomer Royal on Hemiopsy. *London, Edinb. and
   Dubl. Phil. Mag.,* ser. 4, 30:19–21, 1865.
10. Airy, W., ed. *Autobiography of Sir George Biddell Airy.* Cambridge
    Univ. Press, 1896, p. 2.
11. *Ibid.,* pp. 99–100.

Ilza Veith

9

Loneliness and Solitude: Historical and Philosophical Reflections on Voluntary Withdrawal from Society

In solis sis tibi turba locis *(in solitude be your own crowd).*

—Tibullus, *Elegias IV*, xiii, 12

When Greta Garbo arrived in the United States in the early 1930s much of her immediate success was due to her unusual beauty and acting ability; but unique was the mysterious reserve with which she surrounded herself. When besieged by the press she was quoted as saying, "I want to be alone." What she meant was, "I want to be *left* alone." The expressed desire of a beautiful woman to be alone accounts for much of the Garbo mystique: a personality who had the inner resources to find contentment in her own company instead of in the constant presence of reporters and other fawning camp followers of the famous.

It is odd that Americans, usually so sociable and gregarious, were intrigued by a Swedish woman who preferred long solitary walks in unfashionable flat-heeled shoes. For Garbo, far from being censured for refusal to join the crowd, was admired for her social and emotional independence, and while her uncommon beauty added to the mystique, she was venerated for more than being simply a lovely and successful film star. Rather, the mystique was a faint, nostalgic memory of persons who have made solitude a desirable state of contemplation and self-knowledge—those who feel closer to their gods, or their ideals, when they withdraw from society and either establish themselves as hermits or join institutions of withdrawal from the affairs of the world.

In returning to the phenomenon of Greta Garbo and the American reaction to her desire for privacy and solitude, we should note an observation made by many visitors to America: Even now, when newcomers cross the country by train, plane, or automobile, one of the features of the American landscape they find most striking is the enormous distance between human settlements. Outside the large cities, this geographical isolation makes for solitude that is one of the main features distinguishing American life from life in most other Western countries.

Many Europeans consider it desirable to remove themselves from densely populated towns and cherish solitude as a luxury that formerly only great landowners could enjoy. Yet Americans tend to feel uncomfortable in solitude and equate it with rejection; this deprives them of the opportunity for solitary creativity that the European seeks. In this country, a city dweller yearning for solitude may be flattered with the appellation of recluse or eccentric.

The veneration of solitude, widespread in the Europe of the past, evolved from a romanticization of religious beliefs and practices. Many philosophers of the Enlightenment like Rousseau, in his *Reveries d'un promeneur solitaire*—stressed (though they may not really have believed it) that a return to nature and escape from the defiling influence of fellowmen would bring on the intellectually and morally cleansing simplicity characteristic of the first human societies. Even Goethe, who was quite dependent upon human interaction, indulged himself in reveries of the joys of solitude.

For the devout, belief in the desirability of prayerful solitude derived from the pattern of pious ascetics who, like Christ, felt closer to their god in the desert, where their devotion was not deflected by the business of the world. In the third century A.D. Christians eremitical life sprang up in Egypt, where many had fled Roman persecution to live in the desert. Among them, Paul of Thebes was held to be the first hermit. Subsequent establishment of cenobitic (convent) communities and the introduction of rules laid a formal foundation for the institution of monasticism. The word monastery is derived from the Greek *monos*, meaning alone; thus *monastēs* are persons who live in solitude. Monasteries are still "houses of religious retirement," of seclusion from the world for those under religious vows. Besides its philological interpretation, the concept of monasticism carries a connotation of organized asceticism, implying a state of self-imposed self-denial that is carried out towards the achievement of a higher ideal. Not always has monasticism been faithful to this lofty concept.

In most examples mentioned so far, what was chosen was solitude, not spiritual loneliness or isolation. Greta Garbo wanted to be left alone by the interfering representatives of what now are called the Media; part of Jean Jacques Rousseau's work concerns a return to nature. Hermits, monks, nuns, and religious ascetics choose solitude because they believe it will bring them closer to their deity. A revival of much of past striving for solitude may perhaps be found among modern youth, many of whom seek bliss in isolated communes, shacks, and campsites along mountain ranges, rivers, and lakes. Whether they are simply trying out a little reverence for nature, or whether their endeavors will develop into a comprehensive attitude, remains uncertain.

The essays of the French philosopher Michel Montaigne 1533–1592) include one "On Solitude." It reveals Montaigne's intimate knowledge of that state of being: In solitude "Our soul may return to itself; it may keep its own company; it is able to lead an attack, to defend itself; it is able to receive and to give; let us not be afraid to wither in this solitude of monotonous idleness." Then he entreats his readers in the words of Tibullus to find their own crowds in solitude: *In solis sis tibi turba locis.*

A Dutch contemporary unwittingly furnished a living illustration to Montaigne's counsel. The good burghers of Amsterdam were fascinated when the story of a certain hermit appeared in print: The hermit had been a successful Dutch merchant "who gave up his work, in order better to serve his God." Deeply affected by the death of his closest friend, he had moved to the country and was living there in ultimate solitude. When all attempts failed to bring him back to Amsterdam, his former colleagues assaulted him and tried to drag him back bodily. This expression of hostility towards those who are different, especially towards the solitary—the loners or as they are called in German, *die Einzelgänger*—is a general trait. The story of this hermit, like that of most other who chose to live as recluses, does not appear in monastic literature; such individuals, or even groups of individuals, who live a monastery-like existence are regarded as outsiders and amateurs by the monastic "professionals," and as unfair competitors not to be included in official ecclesiastical history.

The distinguished German historian of religion, Professor Ernest Benz, submits an interesting theory of the evolution of eremitism; he considers it concurrent with the history of Western colonization. The hermits preferred solitude to life in the organized church or state; other similarly inclined individuals and even families followed the first hermits, and eventually villages came into being. In this fashion large parts of Italy and Germany were colonized. Similarly, the colonization of Siberia was begun by hermits, who—as nonconformists—had withdrawn from the established church and gradually pushed eastward to set up domiciles. When tax collectors and soldiers arrived, the hermits packed up and moved on.[1]

The history of the eremitical principle has remained scant. Hermits, as a rule, left no traces, for they were not inclined to write autobiographies, or diaries. Nevertheless, it has been possible to piece together a history[2] of the Christian hermit movement up to the late nineteenth century. This movement has by no means expired.

Although one might think that the eremitic movement has no place in Protestantism, studies of the radical pietism of the eighteenth century have uncovered traditions of a hermit-like movement in the Egyptian desert.[3] My own study includes such extremely secluded monasteries as the Greek Orthodox settlement of Mount Athos.

In his work on the Protestant movement towards hermitism, Professor Benz was particularly struck by the realization that it includes the very man whom one would least of all connect with hermitic propensities—Martin Luther. As Professor Benz shows, Martin Luther belonged to the continuum of the old-Christian hermit movement; he entered the hermit branch of the order of St. Augustine after the shattering encounter with a stroke of lightning in which the presence of God was revealed to him. Oddly enough, many students of Luther have assumed that he was a member of the regular order of St. Augustine, whereas in fact he belonged to a separate branch that had been founded centuries before by communities of Italian hermits. Like Luther himself, the medieval founders of these hermit sects had reacted against the feudal aspects of the traditional Roman Catholic Church.

Solitariness and the striving towards eremitical life were distinguishing features not only of some branches of Christianity but also of a number of religious movements originating in the Near East and Far East.

The Coptic Church of Ethiopia arranged for the construction of monasteries on mountaintops that could be reached only by climbing vertical cliffs. The difficulty of access reinforced one of the church's tenets: the total restriction of the monastery to male inhabitants and visitors. So abhorrent was the idea of any kind of female intrusion onto the monasterial mountaintops that only male animals were used for food. Similarly uncontaminated is the Greek Orthodox monastery on top of Mount Athos, which remains inaccessible to females of all species.

Such purity may also be found in some of the Japanese Zen monasteries, although not all Buddhist monastic sects insist on celibacy, and many convents permit monks to have wives and engage in a modicum of family life. Despite current laxity in the matter, the founder of Buddhism left his wife and worldly connections to seek soli-

tude and protection from worldliness as he gave expression to a new
religious belief.

In more recent times, more worldly reasons for withdrawing from society have been mentioned. One prominent spokesman on the subject
was the distinguished physician Johann Georg Zimmermann, whose
four-volume work *Solitude* was published in a variety of editions and
translations in the late eighteenth century.[4] One wonders whether
Zimmermann chose his topic because of his own proclivities to solitude
or whether his own ever-increasing solitariness was the result of his
personality traits and circumstances. At any rate he was beset by
misfortune and increasing loneliness through the deaths of those dear-
est to him. In spite of his professed devotion to the solitude of which
he wrote, Zimmermann expressed the belief that man is born for society and not for a life of withdrawal into loneliness, even if it be
self-imposed. If he felt more and more drawn to that subject, it was
probably because fate had been depriving him of all those who were
essential to his happiness. Almost every association he formed was to
end in his isolation.

In fact, the book requires the reader's complete empathy and
contains little to cheer him. Yet it received such a glowing reception,
especially among the highest social circles of Europe, that Zimmermann was not only appointed personal physician to the King of Hanover, but was even honored by Catherine, the Empress of Russia. Such
a reaction on the part of European royalty strongly intimates the general mood of the leaders of society and the emotional tenor of the period called the Enlightenment. The return to nature, advocated by
Rousseau, implied withdrawal from the business of the world and a
desired solitude in unspoiled surroundings.

The story of Zimmermann's life is typical for a period when man's
life-span was short, when disease was rampant, and when medicine
was far less advanced than it is today.[5]

Zimmermann was born in 1728, in the small Swiss town of Brugg
in the canton of Berne. As was common among children of the European intellectual elite, young Johann Georg received his early school-
ing in all subjects required for admission to the University of Berne
by being tutored by his father, a distinguished and successful elected
member of the Provincial Council. Just before Zimmermann's five years
of philosopy studies at the university, his beloved father died suddenly.
When eventually he gave thought to training in a field that offered a
livelihood, he was again saddened by the death of his mother. In all
probability these two events determined his choice of medicine as a
profession: He wished to be prepared to cope with future illness and

death. As a teacher and model he selected a fellow countryman, Albrecht von Haller, who had achieved extraordinary fame as professor of medicine in the newly founded University of Göttingen. Zimmermann was admitted to that university in the autumn of 1747 and was awarded the degree of doctor of medicine in the summer of 1751.

Impressed with his young disciple, Haller invited him to join his family circle and supervised his postgraduate studies. Zimmermann said that Haller "behaved to him throughout his future life as a parent, a preceptor, a patron, and a friend." Haller's fame had attracted a great many outstanding medical students, among whom Zimmermann stood out as gifted and imaginative. Beyond the mere practice of medicine, he turned his attention to a variety of subjects and found considerable diversion in the study of mathematics, political science, and the new field of statistics. By way of relaxation, Zimmermann learned the English language, and became as conversant with British authors and poets as he was with the German.

But apparently his fervent academic labors had taken their toll of his health, and brought on symptoms of a nervous depressive ailment, then known as hypochondriasis.

To divert his mind and to obtain needed rest and relaxation, he followed a contemporary custom: He took a trip of several months. Unlike other well-born Europeans who traveled to Italy to recuperate under the sun of a southern sky, he sought rest in study and composed an itinerary that would allow him to call on as many celebrated scientists as would receive him. This was an ill-conceived plan. He encountered hostility and competitive tensions among his less successful colleagues in Paris, and suffered a relapse owing to solitary wanderings in a hostile atmosphere. He cured his increasing anguish by returning to Switzerland, where he combined successful medical practice with his former university friends.

While Zimmermann was recovering in Berne, Haller's health also had declined, and he too returned to his hometown for relaxation among his friends and medical advice from his former student, Zimmermann. However, once his health was restored. Haller gave in to the nostalgia, or *Heimweh*, that befalls many Swiss after lengthy absences from home. He decided to resign his professorship in Göttingen, purchased a house in Berne, and sent Zimmermann to Göttingen to assist Haller's family in their move to Switzerland. On that occasion, Zimmermann became attached to Haller's young niece, who lived with the family, and he married her later in Berne.

Now a family man, Zimmermann was offered the position of town physician to his native Brugg and accepted it in spite of the small salary. But the joy of having found recognition in his native city was soon overshadowed by the intellectual limitations of small-town Swiss life. His old school friends represented all the shortcomings of provincial Brugg. When, a few years later, he was offered the position of principal physician to the King of Great Britain, George III, at the court in Hanover, he accepted the appointment with the highest hopes on July 4th, 1768.

But Johann Georg Zimmermann lacked the ability to find and enjoy happiness. He frequently blamed himself for indulging his "saturnine disposition." Yet upon his arrival at the court of Hanover, he found reasons for renewed sorrow. On entering the city gates of Hanover, his carriage overturned, and his mother-in-law, to whom he was particularly devoted, sustained a compound fracture of the leg; she died three days later. Soon after this disaster, Zimmermann began to miss the cordiality of his Swiss colleagues, as his new colleagues in Hanover expressed in all sorts of devious ways their jealousy of his merit and frame. These misfortunes rekindled an old back ailment, and the pain became excruciating. At the same time, the health, of his beloved wife declined and demanded much of his attention. Nevertheless, his medical practice grew in keeping with his professional excellence, and he was kept so busy that he had no chance to give in to his melancholic inclinations. Even his physical pains were subsiding when he was plunged into new and overburdening grief by the death of his wife. In *Solitude,* he philosophized about the inevitable loneliness following the losses he had suffered:

> On the death of a beloved friend we constantly feel a strong desire to withdraw from society; but our worldly acquaintances unite in general to destroy this laudable inclination. Conceiving it improper to mention the subject of our grief, our companions, cold and indifferent to the event, surround us, and think their duties sufficiently discharged by paying the tributary visit, and amusing us with the current topics of the town: such idle pleasantries cannot convey a balm of comfort into the wounded heart.

After this loss, his own painful back condition recurred, and he felt the need to seek medical attention. He went to Berlin and submitted to the care of the famous anatomist and surgeon Meckel, professor at Charité Hospital. Meckel performed such a successful operation that Zimmermann returned to Hanover in a mood of joyful release. In fact, the period of convalescence heralded the happiest time in Zimmermann's life. He had married again, and together with his new wife, enjoyed being the center of the court society of Hanover. But even this period of happiness was clouded by renewed sadness and illness in the family.

His daughter from his first marriage was engaged to be married, but her fiancé, for reasons unknown to all, committed suicide. Upon receiving this shocking news, the girl, who had always suffered from a weak constitution and symptoms of consumption, fell into a "languishing complaint which at length ended in a hemorrhage of the lungs, and in the summer of 1781 destroyed her life."

Even more upsetting was the state of Zimmermann's only son. This young man of uncommon talent fell ill while he was a student at the university and, perhaps weakened by too-intense study, suffered from a worsening of his "bodily infirmity and mental languor which terminated, in December 1777, in total derangement of his faculties, and he continued, in spite of every endeavor to restore him, a perfect idiot for more than twenty years." At the very time of this overwhelming grief, Zimmermann's second wife contracted a severe illness and died.

Zimmermann's private life was now barren of love, but his friends succeeded in finding another wife for the lonely man. This new bride was nearly thirty years younger, "but genius and good sense are always young; and the similarity of their characters obliterated all recollection of disparity of age." More fluent in English than he was, she revised his writings with excellent taste and judgment, and continued to the last moment of her life "his tutelary deity." In her company he enjoyed a more active social life than ever before.

And yet, it was just at this time that he composed his great work *Solitude,* thirty years after the publication of his first essay on that subject. The work was received so favorably throughout Europe that it was expanded from a brief monograph into four volumes and was translated from the original German into French, English, and even Russian. The full title of this work is as cumbersome as the high-flown taste of the period demanded: "*Solitude: or the Effects of Occasional Retirement on the Mind, the Heart, General Society, in Exile, in Old Age; and on the Bed of Death; in which The Question is Considered Whether it is easier to live virtuously in Society, or in Solitude.*"

Europe at that time was very receptive to a work written in a tenor of melancholy. *Solitude* reflected the trend begun by Goethe in 1774, in his immensely successful *Leiden des jungen Werther* (*Sorrows of Young Werther*), which had set the emotional tone; by lending an air of fashion and desirability to explicitly melancholy behavior, it even made suicide an acceptable—and perhaps even admirable—tragedy. In fact, it is quite possible that the seemingly unmotivated suicide of Zimmermann's future son-in-law was a part of the vast wave of suicides that followed the publication of Goethe's work.

Zimmermann himself was scarcely able to tolerate solitude with equanimity for any length of time. But he had an accurate conception of the nature of leisure. He made it clear that leisure is not the same as indolence; rather, it is the interval of relaxation that separates difficulty tasks from pleasant recreations. This sentiment, is an echo of a statement of Publius Cornelius Scipio, who stated that he was never less idle than when he had most leisure, and that he was never less alone than when alone. Zimmermann, on the other hand, emphasized: "Leisure is not to be considered a state of intellectual torpidity, but a new incentive to further activity; it is thought by strong and energetic minds, not as *an end,* but as a *means* of restoring lost activity."

Zimmermann believed that productive solitude could be obtained only in a rural setting, as in the countryside of Switzerland. In cities and towns, productive solitude could be achieved only by withdrawal into one's own study and by exclusion of all disrupting external stimuli; but as he knew from experience, "few men have sufficient resolution to perform it," for even indoors matters of business come up at every moment and interrupt the train of thought.

To continue in Zimmermann's own words:

> Liberty and Leisure are all that an active mind requires in Solitude. The moment such a character finds himself alone, all the energies of his soul put themselves into motion, and rise to a height incomparably greater than they could have reached under the impulse of a mind clogged and oppressed by the encumbrances of society.

In a somewhat unconsciously autobiographical vein he goes on to say:

> Even plodding authors who only endeavor to improve the thoughts of others, and aim not at originality, for themselves derive such advantages from Solitude as to render them contented with their humble labors. . . .

Moreover:

> Solitude encourages the disclosure of those sentiments and feelings which the manners of the world compel us to conceal. The mind there unburdens itself with ease and freedom. The plea indeed is not always taken up because we are alone, but if we are inclined to write we ought to be alone. To cultivate philosophy or court the muse with effects, the mind must be free from all embarrassment. The incessant cries of children, or the frequent intrusion of servants with messages of ceremony and cards of compliment, distract attention.

From these and subsequent thoughts we realize that Zimmermann interpreted the mind as the intellect, whereas the heart represented what present-day language would define as emotion. At the begin-

ning of his discussion of the heart, Zimmermann sums up his feelings
on the mind:

> The highest happiness which is capable of being enjoyed in this
> world consists in *Peace of Mind.* The wise mortal . . . resigns himself
> to the dispensation of his Creator, and looks with an eye of pity on the
> frailties of his fellow-creatures. . . .
> To taste the charm of retirement it is not necessary to divest the heart
> of its emotions.

In the following, Zimmermann further betrays his dependence
upon social response to all his activities and achievements:

> The world may be renounced without renouncing the enjoyments
> which the tear of sensibility is capable of affording.

The most important aspect of the "sensibility of the heart" is the
love of Nature—the love of one's own -country—which in Zimmermann's case (and that of all Swiss) is the love of the Alps:

> Religious awe and rapturous delight are alternately excited by the
> deep gloom of forests, by the tremendous height of broken rocks, and
> by the multiplicity of majestic and sublime objects which are com-
> bined within the site of a delightful and extensive prospect.

Speaking of the value of gardens to the individual, Zimmermann
makes the following observation, which has strikingly modern quality:

> This new re-union of Art and Nature which was not invented in
> *China* but in *England,* is founded upon a rational and refined taste
> for the beauties of Nature, confirmed by experience, and by sentiments
> which a chaste fancy reflects on a feeling heart.

Here the learned Dr. Zimmermann is mistaken, for the fashion in
gardens and their design was actually inspired by the European admiration for *chinoiseries,* which had been introduced through traders
and missionaries posted in China.

He refers to an unnamed English writer who said that "Solitude,
on the first view of it, inspires the mind with terror, because every
thing that brings with it the idea of privation is terrific [terrifying],
and therefore sublime, like space, darkness, and silence."

This terrifying aspect of solitude comes out in certain views of
the Alps, which "appear inconceivably majestic, but on a near approach, they excite ideas certainly sublime, yet mingled with a degree
of terror."

As Zimmermann regarded mundane interruptions of thought as
unavoidable, it is not surprising that his considerations turn to Rous-

seau, who felt miserably impeded in his work at Paris, where the noise of the streets intruded upon his power of concentration.

The remaining chapters of *Solitude* praise retirement over sociability, and indeed maintain that virtue is better served in solitude than in the world. Similarly, even exile can be tolerated if one endures it alone rather than in the company of fellow sufferers.

From this brief summary it may be difficult to understand why this gloomy, repetitious, and somewhat pompous work should have so impressed Zimmermann's contemporaries. The Empress Catherine of Russia, a woman of scientific interests, found the theory of the virtue of solitude so seductive that she sent the author of the treatise an unusual reward: Through the Russian ambassador at Hamburg, Zimmermann was presented with a ring set with a circle of large and lustrous diamonds in the midst of which there was a gold medal bearing the portrait of the Empress. With this the Empress had sent a handwritten dedication: "To M. Zimmermann, Counsellor of State and Physician to his Britannic Majesty, to thank him for the excellent precepts he has given to mankind in his Treatise upon Solitude."

Thus, solitude and loneliness are states of mind rather than reflections of desolate aloneness, and one may feel solitary and alone in the midst of a large gathering of people. As Montaigne said, quoting Horace:

> The savant is able to live everywhere with contentment and is able to be alone even in the crowd of a ducal court; but, if he has the choice, he will avoid even the sight of a crowd. He will, if absolutely necessary, bear the company of a great many people; if, however, it is up to his choice, he will not elect to be in such company. . . .
> The final aim, is always to live in solitude more comfortably and hence more agreeably. Yet one may not always select the right path towards it. Often, one deludes himself to have withdrawn from the business of daily life, when one has only changed it. Moreover, if we have withdrawn from court and business we still haven't freed ourselves from the biggest tormentors of our life: It is reason and wisdom and not a resort hotel by the sea which dissipate our worries. (Horace, Ep. I. xi, 25)

Zimmermann's praise of solitude and his preoccupation with the condition were somewhat inconsistent with his own inability to endure isolation from the stimulating society of his intellectual peers. Nevertheless in considering "the influence of Solitude upon the Mind" he declares: "Solitude teaches one to think, and thought becomes the principal spring of human actions; for the *actions* of men, it is truly said, are nothing more than their *thoughts* embodied and brought into substantive existence." Upon closer reflection these statements reveal a remarkable prescience of later psychoanalytic thought.

It is interesting to note that neither Montaigne, nor Rousseau, nor Zimmermann, nor any of the other religious or lay philosophers of loneliness ever spoke of the search for solitude on the part of women. In fact, the only times women are mentioned in these musings are when it is stressed that the presence of women can only disturb contemplation, and hence solitude.

Except in the setting of the convent whither women might withdraw in the role of nuns, loneliness and solitude were considered contrary to the very essence of woman, whereas certain men were thought to reach their most productive and creative heights in the "private compartment of their own privacy." It is perhaps permissible, therefore, to conclude these reflections with the line of Terence, "Ah, how can any man be convinced that anything is dearer to him as [sic] he himself?"

REFERENCES

1. Ernst Benz, *Evolution and Christian Hope: Man's Concept of the Future from the Early Fathers to Teilhard de Chardin*, transl. by Heinz G. Frank (New York: Doubleday, 1966).
2. H. Guttenberger, *Die Einsiedler in Geschichte und Sage* (Wien: 1928); and W. Nigg, *Vom Geheimnis der Mönche* (Zürich: 1953).
3. Ernst Benz, "Die protestantische Thebais," *Zur Nailer: Nachwirkung Makarios des Aegypters im Protestantismus des 17. und 18. Jahrhunderts in Europa und Amerika,* Akademie d. Wissensch. und der Literatur, Mainz, Abh. der Geistes und der Sozial-Wissensch., Kl. Jg. 1963, Wr. 1. Wiesbaden, 1963.
4. J. G. Zimmermann, *Solitude* (London: Assoc. Book Sellers, 1797).
5. Ibid.

M. Schachter

10

Certainties and Doubts Concerning the Personality and Disease of the Poet Heinrich Heine (1797-1856)

Heinrich Heine, a poet and writer of highest rank in world literature, has long been the subject of study by a great number of literary critics and historians. Furthermore, what is known about the man and the nervous disorder that cut short his life at the age of fifty-nine has not failed to arouse the interest of pathographic investigators.

For critics and historians of literature, there is a considerable body of invaluable source material, composed of the poet's writings and correspondence, and statements from his friends, his intimates, and from some of his editors. Unfortunately, the four volumes of Heine's *Lebenserinnerungen* were destroyed by fire around 1840, so that we possess only a meager text written by Heine in 1854; it was arbitrarily "revised" later by his brother Maximilian, the physician, who took care not to divulge too much intimate information about the family. This text, published in 1883 after the death of the poet's wife Mathilde (née Eugénie Crescence) contained far less than the 160 pages written by its author.

As far as pathographic research is concerned, the available information is both lacunary and scientifically debatable.

This essay concerns a description and diagnosis of the central nervous system disorder that began in 1832 when Heine was thirty-five years old and, after twenty-four years of his suffering, ended in his death in 1856, subsequent to a terminal bulbar impairment. On the basis of particulars furnished by current bibliography, we shall first examine the man Heine and his personality; then we shall seek a medically and scientifically acceptable explanation of the nature of the disease that shortened the poet's life.

As for Heine the man, while deploring the loss of his four-volume memoirs, it is possible, on the basis of the sources indicated, to form a general idea of his life, without the risk of falling into fiction.

The oldest of four children, Heinrich Heine was born in Düsseldorf on December 13, 1791, into a Jewish family whose attitude toward traditional religious practice was somewhat lukewarm, but by no means indifferent.

From his father, a man described as a lover of good living and as a horse fancier who had little aptitude for business, the poet most likely inherited a propensity for worldly pleasure and a rather easygoing nature, combined with something of a contempt for money. A certain frivolity in Heine's nature, in conjunction with a marked sensuality, may perhaps explain the numerous love affairs of the young poet; both in Germany and during his later exile in Paris, he frequented the fashionable salons, where his friendships with women were as varied as his meetings with men whose names were to survive in history.

On the maternal side, the van Gelderns were a family whose culture was at once Jewish and modern. Heine's mother, the daughter of Dr. Gottschalk van Geldern, was well-educated, energetic, realistic; she soon understood her oldest son's artistic and literary talents and helped awaken him to the awareness of his destiny.

A maternal uncle, Simon van Geldern, a cultured and somewhat eccentric bachelor, was the author of works of philosophical, historical, or political pretension, and also probably exerted an influence on young Heine. The same is true, and perhaps even more so, with regard to an older brother of the maternal grandfather, likewise named Simon van Geldern, and known somewhat fancifully as the *chevalier* van Geldern or the "Oriental," on account of his extensive travels in various foreign countries. A *bon vivant* and skirt chaser, this man never attempted to earn any money, preferring to extol his fanatical conception of human liberty. Heine at times termed him a charlatan, while still displaying a certain admiration for him.

His relations, however, were never very close with his paternal uncle, the wealthy banker Salomon Heine, who supplied him with money throughout his life—although Heine considered the amount in no proportion to the uncle's enormous wealth. Nor does the poet seem to have been close to his younger brother, Maximilian, who became a physician. The essential reason for this attitude on the part of the banker and the doctor was perhaps the "ingratitude" of the poet, for they feared his disclosure of "racy" details, especially in his autobiographical writings—and Maximilian was to suppress certain uncomfortable facts.

But while this familial anamnesis throws some light upon Heine's character and temperament—lively, unstable, ironic, sometimes superficial, and a bit megalomaniacal (as when Heine writes to his uncle that it is due to his artistic genius that people talk about "the Heines") —it presents only one aspect of the sensitive, rich, and creative personality of a great poet. For, together with these traits, a rich concatenation of psychological and, above all, political circumstances were to exert a determinative influence upon a large part of Heine's work.

First of all, Heine spent his childhood in a region of Germany that, under Napoleonic occupation, was experiencing for the first time in the history of German Judaism the equality of civil rights conferred by the France of the Revolution. Great hopes were aroused of a better future for Jewish youths, above all for cultured youths. For the already brilliant student, Heine's parents (his mother especially) could envision a career in higher administration or at a university. But the Napoleonic epic came swiftly to an end, and conservative German politics, with its abrogation or limitation of the civil rights granted to Jews, forbade them access to a great number of professions, among them that of teaching in the upper schools and universities.

Heine, who in 1817 at the age of twenty had already begun to publish verses (at first under a pseudonym), enrolled in 1819 under the Faculty of Law at Bonn; he was dismayed and revolted to witness anti-Semitic demonstrations in Hamburg that same year. In 1820, he entered the Faculty of Law at Göttingen, where anti-Semitic feeling ran high; he almost fought a duel with an anti-Semitic student who had insulted him. He left for Berlin; there he attended Hegel's philosophy courses and also frequented the brilliant salons, where his name was beginning to be known.

He quickly realized that life as a Jewish intellectual and a second-class German citizen would be one of inevitable struggle and suffering; moreover, he was financially dependent upon his wealthy uncle, who demanded that he finish his law studies and go into practice in Hamburg. His first publications under his own name and his induction, in 1822, into the famous *Verein für die Cultur und Wissenschaft der Juden* (Society for Jewish Culture and Scholarship) brought him into contact with many personalities; some of them would be his friends for life: Leopold Zunz, Moses Moser, Ludwig Marcus, Lazarus Bendavid, David Friedlander, and Edouard Gans—all writers or scholars whose European culture crowned a thorough knowledge of Judaic history and culture. These significant circumstances in the life of a debutant in the artistic-literary world of the early nineteenth century would, without diminishing any of his affective and emotional inclinations, help to mold the personality of the future great poet.

Having obtained his doctorate in law (*doctor utriusque juris*) at Göttingen in 1825, he followed a trend that was fast becoming an "epidemic" (to use Heine's own term); He converted to Lutheranism, the only way for a Jewish intellectual to gain access to a German university chair. He thought that with this *Taufzettel* (christening certificate), as he was later to call it, he would be able to teach philosophy in Munich or in Berlin. He soon had to resign himself to never obtaining the post he longed for.

It is difficult to believe that Heine, not a believer or churchgoer, converted to Protestantism without having received promises of help in obtaining a post from at least one of his teachers who knew of his brilliance. If he did receive such promises, they were not kept. However, since this very important detail has not been furnished us by any irrefutable document, one is entitled to wonder whether, among other revelations, this one figured in the four incinerated volumes of *Lebenserinnerungen*.

Still, other explanations can be advanced. The university council at Göttingen must have been aware that such conversions often had nothing to do with an authentic change of beliefs. Moreover, we may suppose that certain indiscretions might have revealed that the young poet and doctor of law attached little importance to religion. We know as well that in 1823, two years before his conversion, Heine had written to his friend Moser: "You can deduce from my way of thinking that baptism was not an act of conversion." (This may not have remained unknown.) Only a few months later, he wrote to the same friend: "I am now despised by Christians and Jews. I deeply regret that I was baptized."

However that may be, after his unsuccessful attempt to conduct a law practice, and after new anti-Semitic agitations in Germany, Heine chose exile. In April, 1831, at the age of thirty-four, he arrived in Paris, where he remained until his death.

His decision was certainly not capricious. He was intolerant of that blaze of chauvinistic and anti-Semitic nationalism and clearly saw that he would not be able to write what he wished and as he wished without falling under the blade of a censorship at once severe and stupid.

In the France of Louis-Philippe, Heine found a more breathable atmosphere. He would be able to continue to work and to have his works published in Germany, although the texts were often revised by censors. Moreover, translations into French were continually expanding his influence.

Once more, there were the love affairs and the frequenting of the

Paris salons, where Heine met not only beautiful women but also eminent men in the arts, letters, and even politics. High-strung, passionate, tender, erotic, dreamy, and fanciful, to cite some of the qualities ascribed to him by W. Lange-Eichbaum (to which we may add spendthrift, with no care for the morrow), Heine lived intensely, writing and fighting for a liberal Germany. We know that he was to become fired with enthusiasm for Saint-Simonianism and the ideals of the Revolution of 1848, but that he would be very quickly disillusioned. As a consequence, this admirer of Hellenic civilization, which acclaimed earthly joys, would end up a "Nazarene" (the term is his), in other words, a deist, who, throughout the last years of his life, would proclaim the spiritual superiority of Judaic monotheism. Indeed, in the will drawn up five years before his death, he wrote: "I die in faith in the only God, eternal creator of the universe, whose mercy I implore for my immortal soul."

But to return to 1834, three years after his arrival in Paris: Heine fell in love with the beautiful young Eugénie Crescence (his "Mathilde"), then nineteen years old. Totally uncultivated, Mathilde would be, notwithstanding the spiteful gossip that abounds in certain fictionalized biographies of the poet, a devoted, faithful wife, taking care of her sick husband until the last moment. His illness had begun in 1832; the marriage took place in August, 1844, when Heine was forty-seven years old.

Heine's disease, which progressed slowly, did not prevent him from receiving guests in his home and, perhaps, from loving the beautiful and cultured Madame Elise Krinitz, who wrote under the pseudonym of Camille Selden and whom he immortalized with the name "La Mouche" (The Fly), the insect engraved in her ring.

Of a nature rich but full of contradictions that did not cease to inspire in him works of artistic beauty and biting irony, he had to contend all his life with inelegant shortages of money. Indeed, his incessant requests for money from his wealthy Uncle Salomon run like a red furrow through the poet's life, in his own country as well as in exile in Paris. The reasons for this are hard to understand. It is unlikely that Heine's works, published in both Germany and France, brought in so little as to justify these appeals for help. Rather, since Heine was hyperconscious of his artistic worth yet incapable of managing money, he seems to have squandered everything that he earned or received. That he was neither affectionate nor grateful to the generous uncle contributes nothing to the gilding of the poet's reputation.

Thus, on the intellectual plane as well as on that of artistic sensibility, Heine inherited both the good qualities and the shortcomings of his ancestry, paternal and maternal. He also endured, and in an intense and painful fashion, the political vicissitudes under which Jews lived at that time. His conversion, made solely to obtain a university chair, set off (and not just because he met with failure) feelings of self-depreciation and a deep-rooted aversion to renegades of all times and all places.

Despite all the difficulties and disappointments that filled his short life, Heine still succeeded in creating an imperishable and majestic work.

Let us turn now to the study of Heine as a patient.

To certain men of genius, destiny has shown a cruelty defying human reason. At thirty-five, Heine was intoxicated with the joys of living and loving. His poetic creation was already known and appreciated, but he was tortured by having chosen life in exile, even if he did find this exile more bearable than life in Germany.

Heine would not allow himself to be defeated by his relentlessly progressive and irreversible disease. He continued to work to the farthest limit of his strength.

What was the disease in question?

It was a disorder of the central nervous system that, as far as we know, was neither hereditary nor familial. But what did neurology, as a science, know during the period from 1832 to 1856, the twenty-four years of Heine's illness?

It must be admitted that, in spite of the indisputable and meritorious efforts—as Walther Riese (1959) stresses—of a W. Cullen (1791) and an M. Hall (1841), the meager knowledge of the "morbid anatomy" of the central nervous system, and the *nonexistence* of a histopathology of this same system, did not permit a precise definition, much less an etiological diagnosis, of neurological disorders.

Let us not forget that at the time to which we allude, Charcot was between six and thirty-one years of age and Erb between six and sixteen; that the founder of modern pathological anatomy, R. Virchow, was between eleven and thirty-five years old; that the histopathologist of the nervous system, B. von Gudden, was between eight and thirty-two; or even that Edinger, at Heine's death, was just one year old! In short, the clinical neurology of Heine's day had amassed a great body of information, but it had at its disposal neither a pathological anatomy nor a histopathology worthy of the name.

The onset of the poet's disease has been placed by those who have studied it in 1832, one year after his arrival in Paris. However, some authors have spoken, but without furnishing irrefutable proofs, of frequent headaches going back to adolescence or to his years at the university. We have found no signs pointing to migraine attacks on a heredofamilial basis. Mention has also been made of a syphilitic infection contracted during his student days in Göttingen, but this is probably an assumption based upon the riotous life the young Heine led. In any case, we have no precise information concerning treatments for this disease. What physician would disclose his patients' names, especially in the case of a "secret disease"? Attempts have been made to draw special conclusions from certain confessions of the poet, who (in 1824, at the age of twenty-seven) wrote to his friend Moser, "I have recovered from a bothersome cutaneous affection." This, the Swiss professor Panizza sees as a secondary syphilitic incident, all the more since shortly after the recovery Heine complained of unbearable headaches (with poets, anything will rapidly become "unbearable"). These assertions are invalidated by the poet's long history of such attacks.

It is, therefore, from 1832 on that we have the first trustworthy reports on Heine's slowly progressive neurological disorder, which was treated—to cite the important work of L. Rosenthal—by Doctors Gruby, Sichel, and Wertheim. These physicians did not, to our knowledge, write anything about their illustrious patient.

In 1832, at the age of thirty-five, the poet complained that "two fingers of his left hand were paralyzed"; the clinical examination would show the presence of amyotrophy at that level. Five years later, Heine spoke of his left hand "which grows thinner all the time and is dying." But, at approximately the same time, his physicians noted a mydriasis and disturbed accommodation of the right eye. For defenders of the central neurosyphilitic thesis, this would indicate a mesocephalic impairment by syphilitic arteritis. But rather suddenly and, so it seems, without treatment, these troubles totally disappeared; the poet regained his joy in living and resumed his literary activities.

Was this an infectious neurocentral episode, without relation to syphilitic damage? That would certainly be suggested in our day, and we would, perhaps, be able to look for proof of it, if only by eliminating syphilitic infection.

Heine's respite lasted eight years; in 1845, the eye trouble again appeared. Heine said that he was "about three-fourths blind"; clinically, the physicians observed a bilateral palpebral ptosis. Friends who visited him at the time were struck by a gesture he made almost incessantly: raising his eyelids with his fingers in order to identify those who had come to help him relax. The treatments prescribed (we do not know what they were) did not prevent the generalizing, a year later, of paralysis to almost all the cranial nerves, and in 1847, at the age of fifty, the poet reported noticeable difficulty in walking; his legs were "as if made of cotton" (flaccid paralysis of the lower extremities). "They have to carry me like an infant," he said, with the touch of irony for which he is known. Heine rapidly came to be confined to his bed. The muscular deterioration progressed until, at the age of fifty-two, he was almost totally paralyzed; he could no longer eat without help, and since he also had trouble with the large intestine and the bladder and was complaining of "painful muscular cramps," his physicians were forced to administer opiates.

Despite more and more intensive care, this veritable calvary was to be prolonged for four more years in a patient who retained all his intellectual lucidity. Heine was to suffer repeated attacks of coughing or asphyxia, unquestionably indicatory of bulbar involvement and, hence, of his approaching end. In 1856, at the age of fifty-nine, he was released forever.

Let us stress once more—the statements of his brother, the physician Maximilian, of the physician Gruby, and of Karpeles, the famous German historian of literature, are explicit on this subject— that practically up to the last hour Heine had been able to receive his friends, discuss the problems of the day, laugh, and display his well-known sarcasm as if nothing were the matter. Perhaps we should consider these statements just a bit exaggerated.

Can we actually propose a neurological diagnosis of the disease that struck Heine down?

Diagnoses have been advanced by physician biographers, based on documents or statements. In the perspective of modern neurology, subsequent to Charcot, they have proposed, for instance, an amyotrophic lateral sclerosis, as described by Charcot in 1865, nine years after the poet's death. A. Stern has rejected the hypothesis of polioencephalomyelitis considered by L. Mauthner (1881, cited by W. Lange-Eichbaum) as well as the scarcely credible suggestion of a spinal form of progressive muscular atrophy with terminal bulbar involvement. He follows Hirschler and Lange-Eichbaum in hypothesizing a diffuse cerebrospinal syphilis that, by a curious chance, spared the higher mental functions up to the end. According to Stern, this diagnosis would explain the multiplicity of and fluctuations in the various neurological manifestations: the impairment of the cranial pairs, the sphincter difficulties, and the paralysis and "muscular cramps" from which the poet suffered.

In his recent study of the same problem, K. Kolle thinks that the disease started with an affection of the anterior horns of the medulla (paralysis and atrophy of the left arm), to which were added in succeeding years affection of the oculomotor nerves and those of accommodation. Years later, there occurred impairment of almost all cranial nerves with, in the meantime, flaccid paralysis of the lower extremities, of the bladder, and of the large intestine—the whole being aggravated by diffuse muscular atrophy. In the final stage, this would be a tetraplegia with bulbar paralysis.

According to Kolle, the motor disturbances suggest a diagnosis of progressive spinal muscular atrophy, with terminal bulbar involvement; yet this diagnosis does not tally with the "painful muscular cramps" that made opiates necessary. Was it a matter, perhaps, of a progressive musculoneural atrophy or of a hypertrophic neuritis (Déjerine-Sottas atrophy), which better explains both the disease's onset and the association with atrophic disorders, ocular disturbances, and unbearable pain? Was it a question, perhaps, of a chronic ascending myelopathy of the Landry type? But, in that case, it is difficult to explain the bilateral mydriasis, the paralysis of accommodation, and the affection of the other cranial nerves—a clinical picture that brings to mind a seat at the level of the quadrigeminal bodies.

In attempting to determine the probability of a heredodegenerative disorder (. . . as suggested by the neurologists Kohut, Scheuer, Strodtmann, and Vierordt), Kolle asked the opinion of the neurologist and internist G. Bodechtel, who teaches at the University of Munich. Kolle received the reply that it must be a matter of a cerebrospinal syphilis with impairment of the cranial nerves; hence, not a degenerative disorder. But, once more, why did the patient never exhibit the slightest sign of a mental disturbance? Resignedly, Kolle recognizes that it is impossible, on the basis of the information available, to put forward a satisfying neurological diagnosis.

It seems to us somewhat disturbing to note that there has been no attempt to question whether there was even partially—a pathogenetic connection between the poet's disease and his agitated life, full of conflicts of conscience and of politics.

Some works on psychosomatic neurology based upon the contributions of supposedly profound psychologists (Furtado, R. de Saussure, B. Fernandes) permit one to pose such questions. After all, Tendello (cited by Furtado, 1955) considered that the causality (largo sensu) of neuro-organic diseases was to be sought in a constellation of factors: psycho-organic, somatic, and ecological, acting upon each other and not by the mechanism of simple "arithmetic progression."

Without being able to deny the interest of this clinical analysis, it is obvious that, given the present state of the medical information concerning Heine, we are incapable of pronouncing a scientifically irreproachable judgment.

Our work must not be considered as having been aimed, beyond its strictly scientific objective, at any "recovery" of Heinrich Heine. Heine has no need of champions; his work is known throughout the world. We shall remind his judges of this apothegm from the Talmud: *Sanhedrin sheraouh koulan lekhowah, poutarinn ottho*, that is to say, when a Sanhedrin pronounced a unanimous verdict of guilt, the accused was declared not guilty (*Sanhedrin*, 17, a), as well as the following recommendation from the rabbis: *Hévé dann eth kol haadamm lekhaff zekhout*, you shall judge every man with prejudice in his favor (*Pirkei Avoth*, 1, 6).

REFERENCES

Cohn, M., "Die Krankheit H. Heines," *Deutsche Mediz*, Wschr. 1930.

Keller, W., *Vingt siècles d'histoire du peuple juif* (Paris: Edit. Arthaud, 1971).

Kohn, A., Le déchairement religieux de Henri Heines," *Ass. Méd. Isr. France*, 1953, 45–61.

Kolle, K., "Die Krankheit von Heinrich Heine," *Der Hautarzt*, 15, 1964, 162–164.

Lange-Eichbaum, W., *Genie, Irrsinn und Ruhm* (Müchen-Basel: Edit. E. Reinhardt, 1956).

Riese, W., *A History of Neurology* (New York: M. D. Publications, 1959).

Rosenthal, L., *Heinrich Heine als Jude* (Frankfurt/Main, Berlin et Wien: Verlag Ullstein, 1973).

Stern, A., "H. Heines Krankheit," *Praxis*, 1956, 561–65.

Valentin, A., *Henri Heine* (Paris: Edit. Albin Michel, 1956).

George Mora

11

French Ideology at the Dawn of the American Nation: Cabanis and Jefferson on Psychology and Mental Health Care

The Philosophical Tenets of the Young Jefferson:
His Involvement with the Mentally Ill

In the light of today's attempt to recapture the spirit of life in 1776, one point that deserves consideration is the relationship between the French school of the *Idéologues* and Thomas Jefferson, one of the most illustrious founders of our country, viewed from the perspective of modern psychology. This essay will deal with that relationship and some additional issues that may be of interest to future research.

When Jefferson arrived in Paris as minister to France in 1785, at the age of forty-two, he was exposed to a ferment of philosophical ideas practically unmatched in the Western world since the time of the Greeks. In order to understand the impact these ideas had on him, it is important to review Jefferson's philosophical tenets before his arrival in Paris, as they emerge from available written sources.

The philosophical scene in the United States in the latter part of the eighteenth century—as Riley put it some time ago —was characterized by five main movements: (1) Puritanism from English sources; (2) deism or free-thinking including the revolutionary French skepticism, as a reaction against Calvinism; (3) the idealism of Bishop Berkeley (who had sojourned in Newport, Rhode Island, from 1728 to 1731); (4) Anglo-French materialism; and (5) realism, or philosophy of common sense, from Scotland. "From England came Locke's *Inquiry on Human Understanding*, and Hartley's *Observations on Man;* from France, Condorcet's *Progress of the Human Spirit* and La Mettrie's *Man a Machine;* from Scotland came the similar humanistic treatises of Hume, Reid and Stewart" (Riley).

No one American could combine all these currents into an organic system. In this country, "there was no systematic formulation of human reason—no "Encyclopédie," no "Philosophes," no "esprit de système" (Schneider, p. 35). Yet, "America was then the cosmopolitan frontier in a double sense: It gathered into action the reflections and passions of several generations of European thinkers, and it also led the way toward the bold political, religious, and moral experiments in which the whole world has ever since participated" (Schneider, p. 35). In particular, it was Benjamin Franklin who tried to place the frontier morality on a utilitarian and empirical basis by maintaining the Puritan virtues while abandoning their theological sanctions.

As Chinard has stated in his succinct presentation of Jefferson's philosophy, "The works of the French 'philosophes' had not penetrated very commonly in Virginia" (Chinard, 1943, p. 256). Rather, Jefferson was introduced by his teachers to the works of Bolingbroke, from whom he learned to submit the Bible to historical criticism and was taught to appreciate the classics. In them, and especially in Cicero, he found evidence of the influence of the body on the soul and of the negative influence of the environment on human nature. At the same time, the young Jefferson had found in the Scottish Lord Kames' *Principles of Natural Religion* that the laws of nature could be defined as "rules of our conduct founded on natural principles approved by the moral sense," in other words, the common sense of the common people (Chinard, 1943, p. 258).

Indeed, as another scholar recently put it: "Franklin, like Jefferson, shared many of the concepts of the Scottish Enlightenment. The idea of an innate moral sense was especially appealing . . . [as] a philosophy that would provide support for a belief in an innate moral sense, in the unity of the soul, in freedom of the will, and for a more congenial image of man than the analytical and atomistic one of Locke's sensationalism and Hartley's associationism. (Curti; also Lovejoy, Blau, Nye).

Chinard concluded that "we may safely assume that if, previous to his going to France, Jefferson had become acquainted with the actions of the French 'philosophes,' whatever they may have been, there was very little in these systems which was not equally accessible to him in the works of the ancient philosophers, in the dissertations and disquisitions of the English philosophers, or even in the treatises of the old jurists" (Chinard, 1943, p. 260).

It is plausible that in view of the public offices he held, Jefferson would have been more interested in the practical aspects of human behavior and its aberrations than in the subtleties of the human mind (Hindle, 1956). Actually, he had already been involved with psychiatric issues prior to his arrival in France. On June 4, 1770, a "Bill to make provision for the support and Maintenance of Ideots [sic], Lunatics, and other Persons of unsound Minds" was received and eventually passed by the Virginia House of Burgesses (Dain, p. 9). It provided for the construction of a "public hospital, for the reception of such persons as shall, from time to time, according to the rules and orders established by this act, be sent thereto" (Dain, p. 9). Among the members of a self-perpetuating board or "court of directors" was George Wythe, an outstanding citizen, under whom Jefferson began his apprenticeship in law and whose personal friend he soon became (Dain, p. 10). Eventually, on October 12, 1773, the Asylum was opened at Williamsburg: the first state mental hospital in the United States (Dain, p. 2). Though then very small and able to house only a few patients, it enjoyed a century of renown under the leadership of the Galt family.

In 1777, Jefferson and George Wythe were elected to a committee of five revisors, charged, as he put it, "to take up the whole body of statutes and Virginia laws, to leave out everything obsolete or improper, insert what was wanting, and reduce the whole within as moderate a compass as it would bear, and to the plain language of common sense . . ." (Rutland and Rachal). Jefferson's assignment dealt mainly with the colonial statutes concerning crimes and punishment, religion, and descents (i.e., the law of primogeniture), and with some issues of public education.

By 1779, most of the work had been done by the three lawyer-committeemen (Jefferson, Pendleton, and Wythe). A few bills passed quickly into law, but several years passed before James Madison, at Jefferson's urging, resurrected the ambitious scheme at the May, 1784, session of the General Assembly. While Jefferson was in Paris, Madison took the step of introducing 118 separate bills that had remained from the 126 in Jefferson's original schema. Eventually, 36 bills were adopted, and the one "establishing religious freedom" was coaxed through the General Assembly. However, because of subsequent bureaucratic passivity, to Jefferson's disappointment, the major share of the Revised Code was never enacted into law.

Among the bills presented by Madison on October 31, 1785, and passed by the House and Senate in the following two months, was a "Bill for the Restraint, Maintenance and Cure of Persons not Sound in Mind":

> The present directors of the hospital for reception of persons of unsound minds, and their successors . . . are hereby constituted a body politic and corporate, to have perpetual continuance, by the name of the Directors of the Hospital, for the maintenance and cure of per-

sons of unsound minds; and by that name may sue and be sued . . . and are enabled to take or hold any estate real and personal, given, or to be given, to the said hospital, or to themselves for the use thereof. And the said directors, or any seven of them, the president being one, shall, from time to time, ordain regulations for the government of the said hospital, and appoint a Keeper and a matron thereof, with nurses and guards, when they shall be necessary, and provide for the accommodation, maintenance and cure of the patients remaining and to be received therein. By warrant to be directed to the sheriff, a Justice of the Peace may order to be brought before him any person whose mind, from his own observation, or the information of others, he shall suspect to be unsound and with two other Justices who, at his request, shall associate with him, shall inquire into the state of such person's mind; and the said Justices shall write down as well what shall appear to themselves, as what shall be testified by witnesses, touching the supposed insanity; and, if two of them adjudge the party to be such a one as ought to be confined in the hospital, and some friend will not become bound, with surety, to restrain, and take proper care of him, or her, until the cause for confinement shall cease, the said Justices, or two of them, shall order the insane to be removed to the said hospital, and there received, and from that end direct a warrant to the sheriff, and a mittimus to the said keeper, transmitting therewith to the latter the examinations of the witnesses, and a relation of such facts as the said Justices shall think pertinent to the subject, to be laid before the directors. The said Keeper, immediately after the person removed shall be delivered to him, the receipt of whom he shall acknowledge in a writing signed by him, and given to the sheriff, shall inform the president thereof, who shall require his colleagues to meet as soon as that may be; and at such meeting, which shall not be unnecessarily delayed, the directors, if having considered the case, they concur in the opinion with the Justices, shall register the insane as a patient; but they may, at any time afterwards, deliver him or her to a friend becoming bound to restrain, and take care of him or her, in the same manner as the Justices might have done. If the directors differ in opinion from the Justices, they shall report the matter to the High Court of Chancery, who shall thereupon award the writ de idiota inquirendo, directed to the sheriff of that county, from whence the person supposed to be insane shall have been removed, and such person shall be put into the custody of the said sheriff, and remain there until the inquisition be taken and returned, and then shall be enlarged, or registered, as the said court shall order. The court of a county, city, or borough shall refer it to three Justices to examine into the state of mind of an infant, child, or ward, in their county, city, or borough, suggested to such court, by the parent or guardian, to be insane, and upon the report of the said Justices, if the suggestion appear to be true, shall order such insane to be removed, in the matter before directed, to the hospital, where he or she shall be received and registered. . . . The directors shall enlarge every person confined in the hospital, who shall appear to them to be perfectly cured of insanity, and give such person a certificate thereof. A person registered in the hospital, shall, nevertheless, during the time of his or her confinement there, be deemed an inhabitant in which was his or her legal settlement at the time of his or her removal to the hospital." [Boyd]

The most striking features of this bill appear to be the involvement of the community in the care of the mentally ill, the system of checks and balances to avoid abuses, and in general, the optimistic attitude toward mental illness. Also impressive is the absence of any reference to the role of the physician in mental illness. It is well to note, however, that physicians were by and large not interested in mental disorders at the time and that their number was rather small, especially in the South: Of 312 individuals who received medical degrees before January 1, 1801, only one graduated from William and Mary College (Norwood).

Perhaps more important than this is how the new bill affected the Williamsburg Asylum. What few documents there are indicate that the hospital had to close for some years after the end of the Revolution, and in July, 1781, was in such a short supply of everything that, at the request of the directors, the keeper obtained supplies from the state commissaries through an order of Governor Jefferson, who was then at the end of his term (Dain, p. 22).

Jefferson's direct involvement with the asylum on that occasion is reflected in his *Notes on the State of Virginia*, which appeared in 1785, when he was already in France. "The only public buildings worthy of mention are the capitol, the palace, the college, and the hospital for lunatics, all of them in Williamsburg, heretofore the seat of our government. . . . The college and hospital are rude, misshapen piles, which, but that they have roofs, would be taken for brick-kilns" (Jefferson).

THE SALON OF MME HELVÉTIUS:
THE PHILOSOPHICAL MOVEMENT OF THE IDÉOLOGUES

Before leaving this country in 1785, Jefferson had thus already been influenced by the main tenets of the Enlightenment: the liberal and progressive view of man, and more concretely, a new humanitarian approach to the care of the mentally ill.

Arriving in Paris, Jefferson must have found that these ideas, and many others, were the expression of an entire system of philosophy.

Paris of the late eighteenth century was the cultural center of the universe. All sorts of ideas underlying various philosophical trends were presented in writings by a number of outstanding *philosophes* such as Montesquieu, Rousseau, Voltaire, Turgot, de la Mettrie, d'Holbach, Helvétius, Condorcet, Diderot, D'Alembert. Others, like Buffon, had acquired ample renown for their studies of the natural sciences. Their views were discussed in many salons and literary clubs where the enlightened men of the time (Freemasons, Illuminati, and others) tended to converge. In a more scientific vein, their ideas were debated among the members of august academies, such as the *Académie des Sciences* (1666), or subjected to experimentation in such settings as the *Jardin du Roi* (which later became the *Musée d'Histoire Naturelle*) and the *Observatoire de Paris*. Their writings found their way into the *Journal des Savants* and into other publications that—because of the then universal knowledge of French—were read everywhere (Roger).

But no matter how far-reaching the French thinkers were, their work cannot be separated from that of the British and Germans at a time when the humanistic background based on the classics was still the unifying force among the intellectuals, a force which would lessen only in the mid-nineteenth century. Psychology, in particular, had been influenced by the English thinkers, a fact that undoubtedly contributed to make Jefferson feel somewhat at home during his stay in Paris (Van Duzer; Cailliet; Rosen, 1946; Stein; Manuel; Moravia, 1968, 1970, 1973, 1974).

Also of noteworthy influence was the work of Condillac, who, following British empiricism, attempted to build the entire mental organization of man on sensations, through observation and analysis. In his *Logic* he had stated: "To analyze is nothing but to observe in a successive order the qualities of an object, in order to give them in the mind the simultaneous order in which they exist" (Condillac, 1792). Condillac's philosophical ideas were readily accepted in France and elsewhere because they appeared to offer the epistemological foundation for a number of scientific fields then in the process of renewal; they provided a useful methodological tool for new fields of knowledge, in particular, psychology; moreover, they represented a concrete system devoid of the metaphysical postulates that the generation of the philosophes had opposed without, however, being able to present a viable alternative (Condillac, 1754; 1756; Le Roy; and Knight).

During those decades of the Enlightenment, the various fields of knowledge were still closely connected to each other, and represented by men who were truly humanists. One element that contributed to keep these men together was the social intercourse in the liberal atmosphere of Paris' salons. Of the various salons (which typified the prevailing role of women in the intellectual life of the time) that of Mme Helvétius at Auteuil, near Paris, was the most outstanding. Mme Helvétius' salon has often been mentioned in literature and is the subject of a monograph by A. Guillois written in the past century. At the death of her husband in 1771, Mme Helvétius decided to open the doors of her home, in the peaceful and idyllic surroundings of Auteuil, to a group of outstanding men, who, sharing an interest in liberal thinking and Freemasonry, were soon to constitute the movement of the Idéologues: the litterateur Ginguéné, the economists Say and Roedener, the geographer Volney, the mathematician and cultural historian Condorcet, the physicians Cabanis and Pinel, and last but not least, Benjamin Franklin—to mention but a few.

Franklin, then probably the most famous American, had been in France since 1776, first as a member of the committee to negotiate a treaty and then as a plenipotentiary to France. A resident of the nearby village of Passay, Franklin had become so engrossed with the group of the Idéologues and Mme Helvétius herself that he semi-facetiously asked her to marry him; in spite of her refusal, their relationship remained unchanged until his death in 1790 (Bruce; Van Doren; Aldridge). It was logical that, once arrived in Paris, Franklin would introduce Jefferson to his friends in Auteuil—a true "Académie de Belles Lettres," as he later called it. It certainly would have been more than a challenge for anyone to walk in Franklin's footsteps. Aside from differences in age and in style—the Quaker Franklin versus the Southern aristocratic Jefferson— Franklin represented the world of the passing Ancient Régime while Jefferson represented the new and revolutionary spirit that was soon to sweep the country. Yet, endowed with that natural aristocracy of which he was fond, Jefferson accepted the challenge and soon felt at ease among the Idéologues (Picavet).

An exciting spirit of a genuine search for knowledge permeated that group. At the time of Jefferson's sojourn in Paris, the various intellectuals gathering at Auteuil were in the process of applying Condillac's method to the study of the mind. This does not mean that they passively accepted his philosophical postulates, but they certainly accepted his method of analysis, from which a new synthesis emerged. However, they also became progressively aware of Condillac's shortcomings: his basic dualistic Cartesianism, his disregard for physiology, and his uncritical philosophical reduction of everything to a single principle.

Destutt de Tracy, another Idéologue, had essentially accepted Condillac's tenets on sensation. As George Boas put it years ago: "The only difference he finds between thinking and feeling is one of time. Sensations which are no longer in process of production are thought; while they are being produced, they are felt. But the material of consciousness is absolutely homogeneous—it is perception of sensations. All this material naturally comes to us through our sense organs." Yet Destutt de Tracy, in his writings, had also advocated the empirical method of analysis, the realistic modification of Condillac's sensationalism and the importance of activity and will as the bridge between knowledge and society. In the "reunion of our faculty of willing, with that of moving ourselves, and feeling," a method emerged of treating ideas by reducing them to original feelings, activity, or sensation. Ideology was thus a method for investigating the instruments and results of human knowledge and for placing on a concrete basis the fields of morality, economics, and education, at variance with the traditional emphasis on reason and authority.

Whether focusing on analysis or on observation, the main theme of the Idéologues remained that of the *science de l'homme.* No matter how appealing all this must have been to the author of the *Notes on the State of Virginia,* it was the application of ideology to the study of man, anticipating a new and real anthropological approach, that captured his strongest and sustained interest.

This new approach was propagated by Cabanis. Who was Cabanis? Born in 1757 in southwestern France, he had attended a religious school and then, at fourteen, had immersed himself in the study of physics and logic in Paris. Secretary to the prince-bishop of Wilna, Poland, at eighteen, he returned to France two years later and studied medicine, graduating in 1784. In 1778, he was introduced to Mme Helvétius' salon. Seeing a resemblance to a lost son, she adopted him, and he remained with her for the next thirty years, almost to the end of his life (Poyer; Gouhier; Lehec; Canguilhem). The years between 1785 and 1789—which coincided with Jefferson's stay in Paris—were for Cabanis a period of intense work. He completed his *On the Degree of Certitude in Medicine* (1789) and *Essay on Public Education* (1791). Endowed with an extremely appealing personality and high intelligence, Cabanis soon elicited the respect and admiration of all those attending the salon of Mme Helvétius, including Franklin and Jefferson.

During that period, Cabanis was already working on the theme of the relationship between the physical and the moral aspect of man, which resulted in his famous "Mémoires." Widely read after 1796, they were published in 1802 as *Rapports du physique et du moral de l'homme.* Contrary to traditional metaphysics and to speculations about ultimate causes, Cabanis emphasized the observation of the phenomena themselves, the order in which they occur and their reciprocal relationship, and the importance of classifying them so that they represent that order and relationship. His biological determinism was thus progressive and hierarchic. For him, the study of the physical aspect of man was paramount both for the physician and the moralist. In fact, moral life could not be considered separate from organic existence; rather, it signified an essential element of the human being. Cabanis' masterpiece represents a continuous interfacing between the organic elements and the moral and intellectual aspects of human life. Medicine and morality are for him two aspects of the same science: the "science of man." As he put it: "physiology, analysis of ideas, and morality, are nothing but three branches of a single and same science which can be rightly called 'Science of man'; i.e., what the Germans call 'anthropology'" (Cabanis, 1804).

From Condillac on, sensibility had been based exclusively on the perception of the external reality through the various senses. Now, Cabanis claimed that there were two other sources of sensibility: one resulting from the nervous system itself, the other resulting from the functioning of the internal organs, both unconscious and both apt to become conscious only when they were increased in pathological conditions. Moreover, such a sensibility had to be viewed from a developmental as well as an environmental perspective.

Nothing is less true than to assume that the human being at birth is devoid of sensations and feelings. Rather, the newborn is affected by sympathy, the fundamental tendency of human nature, which determines the way in which the various sensations and feelings are connected with each other. The newborn, before being subjected to external stimuli, already has tastes and tendencies; reminiscent of some animals that try to use certain parts of the body before they have reached a proper stage of development. In the human being, the various instincts (from the Greek for "to stimulate inside") develop according to the predominance of the various parts: "The brain and heart develop the instinct of conservation; the digestive tract enhances the instinct of nutrition; and the muscular system is responsible for the instinct of movement.

Needs and states of mind depend on the conditions of the internal organs, which are different at different ages. In particular, ideas and feelings related to the development of sexual organs depend on internal impressions. Such impressions are further influenced by the particular temperament of each individual: sanguine, melancholic, phlegmatic, and choleric (the famous four temperaments of Greek medicine), to which Cabanis added the nervous and the muscular ones. Moreover, environmental factors of all kinds, in particular the regime and the climate (as already emphasized by Hippocrates) influence the human being. Life, for Cabanis, is ruled by the law of attraction. Every being has a center of gravity, around which by attraction similar elements gather and dispose themselves hierarchically according to their nature and their reciprocal relationship. The nervous system, as he conceived it, results from the combination of various lower systems, each one centered around a partial "ego." Yet, the human being is a living unity, a functional harmony, that can be subjected to analytic study (Poyer, 1910).

In the field of psychiatry, Cabanis offered in the tenth memoir of his *Rapports du physique et du moral de l'homme* four types of disorders or main causes for the occurrence of insanity: (1) sensations proper related to the contact of the nervous system with the external world, of which the sense of touch is paramount; (2) sensations received by the inner nervous extremities, particularly those innervating the digestive system and the sexual organs; (3) impressions occurring in the matter of the nervous system itself; and (4) instinctual tendencies, desires, and urges related to the three factors mentioned above, caused by action of *sympathies*.

The illusions and the sensorial and cenesthetic hallucinations of today's psychopathology were to be attributed to these four types of disorders. Impressions deriving from the nervous system itself were to explain the occurrence of insanity, epilepsy, and ecstasy, as well as of sleep. It was Cabanis' hope that the refinement of the anatomo-pathology of the central nervous system would eventually lead to uncovering the etiology of many cases of insanity. Moreover, in a number of cases, remedies for a physical illness had brought about the disappearance of related mental disorders.

To be sure, not all cases of mental disorders were explainable on an organic basis, and many cases of insanity had to be explained on a functional basis. As a matter of fact, it seems appropriate to use the study of abnormal psychological phenomena to explain normal psychological phenomena. In particular, dreams present many similarities to delusions and are related to the conditions of the intestinal tract, of the sexual organs, and of other systems—the dream appears to be a delusion in the state of sleep, and the delusion a dream in the state of wakefulness (Genil-Perrin, (a) 1920).

Even from this brief sketch of Cabanis' ideas, it is clear that he anticipated current notions of the unconscious, of cenesthesia, of instinctual urges, of psychosomatic medicine, and in general, of the unit of the personality. It is, therefore, hard to understand that his name has passed largely unnoticed. Probably two factors have contributed to this neglect: the rejection by the masters of the French Restoration

(1815–1830) of his work as materialistic and atheistic (especially because of his famous pronouncement that thought is the secretion of the brain); and his position of *médecin-philosophe,* which may have prevented him from being accepted by either the physicians or the philosophers (Gusdorf). Whereas years ago only a few knew him as the founder of physiological psychology (Poyer, 1910) and scientific psychology (Genil-Perrin), today he may be considered one of the most important precursors of dynamic psychology, as well as "the best known philosopher of the medical revolution" (Ackerknecht, p. 3) and the successful achiever of a "synthesis between ancient stoicism and the eighteenth-century empiricism" (Cazeneuve).

CABANIS AND PINEL:
THE INFLUENCE OF THE IDÉOLOGUES ON THE REFORM OF THE TREATMENT OF THE MENTALLY ILL

Cabanis's pioneering role reforming the treatment of the mentally ill has been as much neglected as his innovating concepts in psychology. In fact, the credit for employing more humane methods of restraint in the treatment of the mentally ill usually goes to Philippe Pinel (1745–1826). The dramatic scene of Pinel liberating the mentally ill from their chains at Bicêtre in 1793, and two years later, at the Salpêtrière (as immortalized in the painting by Robert Fleury), has been reprinted in many psychiatric books. It is less known, however, that Cabanis was instrumental in getting Pinel appointed at Bicêtre. To understand the significance of Pinel's gesture and, even more, of his "moral treatment," it is important to know the attitude toward mental illness in eighteenth-century France.

The era of the Enlightenment has been characterized by great conflict between conservative and progressive forces. While advances were made in all fields, including the study of the mind (e.g., the fine psychological analyses of the English empiricists and the French moralists), the mentally ill remained neglected. To the adherents of the Protestant ethic, for whom labor became equated with morality and idleness with sin, the mentally ill seemed taken care of; they were kept in large institutions (like the Hôtel-Dieu in Paris), which were a combination of penal reformatory, insane asylum, sheltered workshop, and hospital, where paupers, vagrants, defectives, epileptics, and the crippled were also housed (Richmond).

The justification for the "great confinement"—as this trend has been labeled by M. Foucault (1965)—lies in the glorification of reason and the condemnation of the irrational, in line with the rationalistic philosophy of the eighteenth century. The fear of madness, perhaps influenced by the idea of contagion resulting from the new concern for public health, appeared to have replaced the fear of plague or, earlier, that of leprosy. The mentally ill were the subject of much abuse and ridicule, and were carefully avoided by most of the physicians.

Slowly, however, toward the end of the century, a new social conscience started to develop (McCloy), and ideas for a more enlightened treatment of the mentally ill began to emerge. The physician Jean Colombier (1736-1789), general inspector of hospitals and prisons in France, published in 1785 a report entitled "Instructions on the manner of governing the insane, the proper characteristics of the establishments which receive them, the diet and the medical service." In it he exposed the neglect of the communities toward their mentally sick members and the abuses and cruelties that took place in the institutions that housed them. He advocated kind treatment for the mentally ill, a good number of whom could regain reason, and suggested that patients be divided into groups according to their condition. Ideally, they should be cared for in individual beds in an institution located in the country (Semelaigne, (a) 1930).

Three years later a report appeared by Jacques-René Tenon (1724–1816), then surgeon at the Salpêtrière, in which he disclosed the horrible conditions of the inmates of the Hôtel-Dieu (Semelaigne, (b) 1930). In the following year the French Revolution exploded. Among those elected to the *États-Généraux* in 1789 was the Duc de Larochefoucauld-Liancourt (1747–1827) (Dreyfus). The following year the *Comité de Mendicité,* a sort of Committee on Welfare, was established by the National Assembly under Larochefoucauld-Liancourt's presidency. This committee surveyed all welfare facilities, especially those of large institutions such as the Hôtel-Dieu, Bicêtre, and Salpêtrière, gathered data about the treatment of the mentally ill abroad (including the United States), and submitted a plan for a network of welfare facilities, including two hospitals for the treatment of insanity ("the disease most afflicting and humiliating for mankind, whose cure offers the greatest satisfaction to the mind and the heart" [Dreyfus, p. 161]), one private institution similar to the York Retreat, and one public asylum for the incurable.

In 1791, Cabanis was named a member of a five-man *Commission des Hôpitaux,* charged with the reorganization of the hospitals, especially in Paris. The year before, with Tenon's work as an example, he had published a short tract, called *Observations sur les Hôpitaux,* in which he advanced all kinds of suggestions for improving the hospital system, and in particular recommended the replacement of large with small hospitals, in view of the difficulty of treating furious maniacs in large settings.

A few years later, Cabanis published a summary of various reports made to the *Commission des Hôpitaux* (Cabanis, 1793), in which he recommended that only the truly mentally ill pauper should be accepted in public institutions to avoid unnecessary crowding. In the spirit of the French Revolution, he stated that "it is the freedom, it is the safety of people that we have to provide before anything else" (Cabanis, 1798–1800). As much as possible, he wrote, the mentally ill should remain in the care of his family. As mental illness is not irreversible or incurable, the physician should decide on the treatment and consider the possibly dangerous behavior of the patient. Issues related to the commitment of the patient, he felt, were of pertinence to the legal authorities. To keep the patient active through a well-designed regime of work would be essential in most cases; many of them could then return to their families and the community. For those who needed restraint, the best method would be the straitjacket as employed in the English hospitals.

Influenced by the revolutionary ideals, Cabanis concluded by saying that:

> . . . under the effect of wise institutions which constitute a true Republic, insanity and all disorders of the mind will eventually become less frequent. Society does no longer degrade man . . . the customs of ignorance, derision, misery will no longer surround man from the cradle on. Subjected only to the necessary evils of nature, man will be spared the disorders of the mind which are directly caused by a faulty social situation and, consequently, the unfortunate consequences that such a situation elicits. Finally, the moment will come when perhaps the only cause of insanity will be the congenital abnormality of the bodily organism or the unforeseeable accidents of human life which no wisdom can prevent.

Needless to say, such a vast program of prevention, utopian even in our days, could not be accomplished at that time. But Cabanis did accomplish one very important thing: Together with his colleague Thouret of the *Commission des Hôpitaux,* he proposed Pinel for the position of physician at Bicêtre. In spite of an initial reluctance, Pinel eventually accepted and was named to that position in 1793; Cabanis finally had an opportunity to see the tenets of his ideology applied to mental illness.

When Pinel arrived in Paris in 1778, he had already been exposed to the classical concepts and English liberal thought. Thanks to a friendship with a medical student from England during his studies at Montpellier, he became fluent in English (Lechler). In Paris, Cabanis soon introduced him to the salon of Mme Helvétius, where he met several of the Idéologues, including Benjamin Franklin. The suicide of a young man to whom Pinel was close seems to have turned him toward the study of mental diseases. He may himself have suffered a spell of depression after a second failure to obtain a prize to become *médecin regent;* a failure that his biographers attribute to his timidity. It was at that time, probably at Franklin's suggestion, that he seriously considered the possibility of emigrating to the United States—an idea he finally abandoned by the end of 1784.

That same year he accepted an invitation to translate William Cullen's *Institutions of Medicine* and to summarize the *Philosophical Transactions of the Royal Society*: Both these works contained references to mental illness and its treatment. He also began to edit the *Gazette de Santé*, in which he published a number of articles related to mental illness (Semelaigne, 1888, 1912). As a result of several years of experience gained at the Maison Belhomme, a small private mental institution (Bernard), he reported on the "moral regime which is the most appropriate for re-establishing in certain cases the distraught reason of maniacs" (Chabert).

In his many publications on Pinel, Walther Riese has investigated more thoroughly than anyone else the influence of Hippocrates and the Idéologues on Pinel (Riese, 1966, 1968, 1969; and especially *The Legacy of Philippe Pinel*, 1969). With the help of these studies, as well as those by Rosen, Ackerknecht, and others, it is now possible to state that Pinel was mainly influenced by Locke and other empiricists, either directly or through Condillac's most important work, *Traité des Sensations* (1754). In the paper "Research and observations on the moral treatment of the insane," published in 1799, Pinel remarked: "Can one describe the symptoms of insanity if one has not analyzed with Locke and Condillac the functions of human understanding? . . . So I had to retrace my steps and study the writings of our modern psychologists, Locke, Harris, Condillac, Smith, Stewart."

Stewart was, of course, Dugald Stewart, one of the main representatives of the Scottish philosophy of common sense; Smith was evidently Adam Smith, who was associated with Helvétius, Turgot, and Quesney during the time he lived in Paris. Pinel undoubtedly heard of him in Mme Helvétius' salon, since a friend of hers, Mme de Condorcet, had translated Smith's work, and it is her version that he cites in his *Traité*. Indeed, in the introduction to his *Traité médico-philosophique sur l'aliénation mentale ou la manie* (1801), Pinel again spoke of his intellectual debt to Locke and Condillac.

It is likely that Cabanis and Pinel influenced each other reciprocally. Certainly both men were equally concerned about the state of medicine. Medicine was then torn between the mechanistic trend of iatromechanics and iatrophysics on the one side, and the vitalism of the school of Montpellier and the German Stahl on the other side—both unable to provide a concrete and meaningful approach to the study of man (Moravia, 1972; King).

As has been pointed out, the interplay between medicine and philosophy represented a fruitful approach to a theoretical foundation of medicine; the rediscovery of Hippocratic themes, however, provided a practical approach to the study of the clinical syndromes and the treatment of the individual patient. Cabanis' already-mentioned *On the Degree of Certitude in Medicine* (1789) and Pinel's *Philosophical Nosography or the Method of Analysis Applied to Medicine* (1798), constituted the most mature application of ideology to medicine. Indeed, even in his treatise on mental illness, Pinel had based his psychopathology (notably in the study of memory and of intelligence) on ideology, (Colonna d'Istria; Woods and Carlson; Grange; Mackler and Bernstein).

So, in a few years, a handful of *médecins-philosophes* in Paris created a new school of medicine based on clinical observation which soon became well known the world over (Rosen, 1956; Jetter; Weiner; Foucault, 1973; Ackerknecht). The *Société Royale de Médecine* (founded by Vico D'Azir in 1776) and the *Société Médicale d'Emulation* (founded in 1796 by Corvisart, Bichat, and others) were to gather the most important medical minds of the time. In retrospect, of the médecins-philosophes, Cabanis represented the theoretician, Pinel the practitioner. Cabanis died at the age of fifty-one unable to complete a study on the moral improvement of mankind, for which he had prepared a considerable amount of material. Pinel, on the other hand, was able to carry on his reform for another three decades, surrounded by a group of distinguished pupils who were to constitute the French school of psychiatry. Thus, his figure has come to overshadow that of Cabanis.

THE IDÉOLOGUES AND JEFFERSON
AFTER HIS RETURN TO THE UNITED STATES

The Rise and the Decline of the Idéologues

Jefferson's return to the United States was followed by a period of intense work as Secretary of State from 1790 to 1793. Although he found it difficult, at times, to keep in touch with his French friends because of the pressure of his work, his ties to them remained strong for the rest of his life. A year after Franklin's death he sent a message to the president of the French National Assembly to express the appreciation of Congress for the Assembly's decree of June 11, 1790, honoring Franklin's memory (Chinard, 1955).

Conversely, Franklin's and Jefferson's involvement with the circle of Auteuil was to have a significant impact on the guests of Mme Helvétius. Franklin and Cabanis had developed a kind of father-son relationship. Sometime between 1798 and 1800, Cabanis wrote a *Notice sur Benjamin Franklin,* in which he emphasized the importance of the latter's social and humanitarian work.

Indeed, the example of the United States as a new country embracing liberal and republican ideals had had a strong effect on the theoretically inclined minds of the Idéologues. The fact that for the first time in history these ideals were applied in a peaceful and enlightened way could not fail to impress them. Jefferson had translated these ideals into the *Declaration of Independence.* The example of the Americans was destined to have repercussions among the guests at Auteuil. It is possible, therefore, that Franklin's many educational and social endeavors moved Cabanis to concern himself with the reorganization of schools, hospitals, and other social institutions to the point where his early writings reflected the sociological and even political concerns more than the medical.

The year of Jefferson's return to the United States, 1789, coincided with the beginning of the French Revolution. It was also the end of the first period of splendor of the salon d'Auteuil, notable for the transition from the philosophes to the Idéologues, and for the strong belief in the possibility of a peaceful renewal of society.

With the death of Mirabeau—who had been treated by Cabanis (Cabanis, 1791)—and the arrest of King Louis XVI, the work of the Constituent Assembly terminated and a new era dawned for France, marked by disorder and rebellion. As the Idéologues could not help but be opposed to violence in politics, they soon came to be prosecuted by Robespierre during the Reign of Terror. Many of them, including Destutt de Tracy, were jailed; Condorcet committed suicide with a poison given to him by Cabanis, who remained in seclusion at Auteuil. It was at that time that Cabanis, probably on Jefferson's suggestion, was offered the position of Minister of France to the United States. Cabanis was no stranger to the United States, having been elected a member of the American Philosophical Society in 1786 (Rosengarten). He declined the position, however, because of his ties with Mme Helvétius and, even more, with Charlotte Grouchy, the sister-in-law of Condorcet, whom he eventually married.

The years from 1794 to 1799 represent a second period of splendor for the group of the Idéologues. In the confusion that followed

Robespierre's fall, many turned to the Idéologues for leadership and guidance in social, educational, and scientific matters. Some became members of a commission charged with formulating a new constitution; almost all contributed to the magazine *Décade Philosophique* (1794–1807). At the newly created *Institut National,* one section (*section de l'analyse des sensations et des idées*) was completely devoted to ideology. In 1799, Cabanis was named professor of legal medicine and subsequently professor of history of medicine, though he never taught because of poor health.

During that same year, Napoleon shaped a *coup d'état* that resulted in the dissolution of the Council of the Five Hundred (of which Cabanis had been a member since 1797), in the overthrowing of the Directory, and, eventually in his nomination as First Consul. Like the other Idéologues who were convinced of the need of political support for the spread of their ideas, Cabanis actively supported Napoleon and even gave a speech at the Council of the Five Hundred the day after the coup. Napoleon was then considered close to the Idéologues, having been introduced to the society of Auteuil in 1795.

So, for the third time, the Idéologues were involved in political action. Cabanis was charged with the preparation of a political project leading to a new constitution, an indication of the prestige in which he was held. Elected to the senate, he became—as Moravia (1968) put it—"the theoretician of the new consular regime."

Nowhere was the influence of the Idéologues more noticeable in that period than in education, to the point that the educational reforms then under way in France were responsible for a new chapter in the history of education in Europe. Cabanis, again, played a central role in this movement, with his *Travail sur l'éducation publique* (1791), in which the aim of education, a new kind of man, viewed from the ideological perspective, was clearly stated. (A number of concrete proposals presented in this work were implemented by the newly established *Comité d'Instruction Publique,* in which Cabanis was also involved.) Essentially, this movement held that republican ideals could be achieved only in a nation where public education was widespread. Moreover, specialized personnel should be trained for the tremendous political and social endeavors that France was then carrying on in Europe and elsewhere. Ideology, thus, became a basic subject of teaching and was, in line with Destutt de Tracy's philosophy, taught as "general grammar," especially in the newly formed *Ecoles Centrales* (Taton; Gillispie, (a), (b); Fayet).

It was inevitable, however, that a conflict should arise between the enlightened philosophy of the Idéologues and Napoleon's progressively dictatorial trends, as evidenced by the reorganization of the

Institut National in 1802, with the resulting elimination of the above-mentioned *section de l'analyse des sensations et des idées*. Napoleon, unable to attract the Idéologues to his side, developed an increasing aversion to them; conversely, the Idéologues, disappointed in their expectations, withdrew from public life. Cabanis, already failing in health, remained for long periods at Auteuil and then moved to Rueil, where he died in 1803.

Correspondence between Jefferson and the Idéologues

There is little doubt that Jefferson kept himself informed about the major developments that were affecting the most important members of the société d'Auteuil, and specifically in regard to Cabanis, whose two volumes of *Rapports du physique et du moral de l'homme* had first appeared in 1802. In the same year Cabanis sent a copy of them to Jefferson, accompanied by a letter that said in part:

> I am taking the liberty of offering you a copy of a work which I have just published in France, and whose topic constitutes the thorough basis for moral sciences. Being aware of the many things which occupy you, I certainly do not expect that you will have the time to read two massive volumes; I hope, at least, that you will be disposed toward this sincere token of my admiration and respect for you. I trust that you will not have forgotten the persons who had the experience of knowing you at the home of the wonderful Mme Helvétius, and the famous doctor Franklin. We have lost Mme Helvétius; and the citizen La Roche and I now occupy the home according to her will—a very touching disposition inasmuch as her remains lie in the yard. It is there, Mr. President, that I had the pleasure of meeting you some times; it is there that after your departure for America we have so often talked about you with that venerable friend. [Chinard, 1925]

Upon receiving the two volumes, Jefferson wrote him the following on July 12, 1803:

> Dear Sir—I lately received your friendly letter of 28 Vend. An. XI, Oct. 20, 1802 with the two volumes on the relations between the physical and moral faculties of man. This has ever been a subject of great interest to the inquisitive mind, and it could not have got into better hands for discussion than yours. That thought may be a faculty of our material organization, has been believed in the gross; and though the "modus operandi" of nature, in this, as in most other cases, can never be developed and demonstrated to beings united as we are, yet I feel confident you will have conducted us as far on the road as we can go, and have lodged us within reconnoitering distance of the citadel itself. . . . It is with great satisfaction, too, I recollect

the agreeable hours I have passed with yourself and M. de la Roche, at the house of our late excellent friend, Madame Helvétius, and elsewhere; and I am happy to learn you continue your residence there. Auteuil always appeared to me a delightful village, and Madame Helvétius the most delightful spot in it. In those days how sanguine we were! and how soon were the virtuous hopes and confidence of every good man blasted! and how many excellent friends have we lost in your efforts towards self-government, "et cui bono." . . . [Lipscomb, vol. 10, p. 104]

Later on, in a letter of February 8, 1805, directed to the French philosophe and historian, C.F.C. de Volney (the author of the then-famous *Voyage en Egypte et en Syrie* [1787], who lived in this country from 1795 to 1798), Jefferson wrote: "I am glad to hear that M. Cabanis is engaged in writing on the reformation in medicine. It needs the hand of a reformer, and cannot be in better hands than his" (Lipscomb, vol. 11, p. 68). On July 10, 1812, in a letter to Thomas Cooper, Jefferson said that "Tracy should be preceded by a mature study of the most profound of all human compositions, Cabanis' *Rapport du physique et du moral de l'homme*" (Lipscomb, vol. 13, p. 177). Cooper, then president of South Carolina College, wrote Jefferson on May 31, 1814: "I have been reading very carefully, with great interest and instruction the work of Cabanis. . . . Cabanis had boldly drawn the unavoidable conclusion, which Hartley was obliged to compromise about. . . . I should greatly like to translate Cabanis, but I fear the public would not bear it. Too much light is apt to blind us" (Lipscomb, vol. 13, p. 177). In a letter to John Adams of March 14, 1820, after having expressed admiration for Destutt de Tracy, Jefferson says that "Cabanis, in his *Physique et morale de l'homme,* has investigated anatomically, and most ingeniously, the particular organs in the human structure which may most probably exercise that faculty" (Lipscomb, vol. 15, p. 240). Finally, already octagenary, in 1825, in a thankful note to Lafayette upon receiving Flourens' book on the functions of the nervous system in the vertebrate animals, Jefferson said: "Cabanis has gone far towards proving from the anatomical structure and action of the human machine that certain parts of it were probably the organs of thought and consequently that matter might exercise that faculty" (Lipscomb, vol. 19, p. 281).

Although Cabanis' main work was not translated into English, another work by him, *An Essay on the Certainty of Medicine,* had appeared in Philadelphia in 1823, translated by R. de la Roche, M.D. (Was he a relative of the Idéologue Abbé de la Roche, of whom Jefferson spoke so warmly in the correspondence quoted above? [Chinard, 1925]) It is likely that Jefferson was somewhat involved in this translation, a copy of which is in the catalogue of the Library of Congress, whose nucleus consisted of Jefferson's library.

Cabanis' focus on the concrete study of human behavior, either moral (i.e., psychological) or physical, as a foundation for a unified science of man, may have had particular appeal to Jefferson. He, too, put the emphasis on individuality, as shown in a letter to Dr. Manners of February 22, 1814: "Nature has, in truth, produced units only through all her works. Classes, orders, genre, species, are not of her work. Her creation is individual. No two animals are exactly alike...." (Lipscomb, vol. 14, p. 143). And, elsewhere: "Men living in different countries, under different circumstances, different habits and regimes, may have different utilities; the same act, therefore, may be useful, and consequently virtuous in one country while it is injurious and vicious in another differently circumstanced" (Lipscomb, vol. 14, p. 143).

To the end of his days, Jefferson admired the school of the *Idéologues*. As a matter of fact, he managed to have two of Destutt de Tracy's main works appear in English translation in this country: *A Commentary and Review of Montesquieu's Spirit of Laws* in Philadelphia in 1811 and *A Treatise on Political Economy* in Georgetown, D.C., in 1817. As A. Koch relates, "In America ideology was introduced solely through Jefferson's efforts in its behalf and was confined almost exclusively to the writings of Tracy, with some attention to Cabanis and J. B. Say." This was echoed by George Rosen's statement that "Jeffersonian thought may thus be considered in part, at least, as an extension of Ideology to the American scene." (Rosen, 1952)

Jefferson's Contact with European Emigrés

Aside from their correspondence with Jefferson, many American intellectuals seem to have been influenced by the Idéologues, either through their works or through their contact with French immigrants. As demonstrated by Howard Mumford Jones fifty years ago (Jones, p. 151) and more recently by others (mainly Echeverria), the French influence on this country during the late eighteenth and early nineteeth centuries was apparent in social manners, art, religion, and politics. Voltaire's and Rousseau's main works as well as Condorcet's *Progress of the Human Spirit* and La Mettrie's *Man a Machine*, were read and discussed frequently.

Even more important, many ideas of the Idéologues may have been introduced here by some of the *émigrés* fleeing the horrors of the French Revolution. Outstanding among them was the Duc de Larochefoucauld-Liancourt, already mentioned in his role as presi-

dent of the *Comité de Mendacité* (Dreyfus). An enlightened philan-
thropist not closely connected with the Idéologues, he had attempted
to act as the intermediary between King Louis XVI and the Assembly,
of which he had been elected president. In 1789, following an order
for his arrest, he had escaped to England, and in 1794 emigrated to
America.

As a result of his travels throughout almost all the Atlantic Coast
states and Canada, in 1799 Liancourt published his *Voyage dans les
Etats-Unis d'Amerique fait en 1795, 1796 et 1797*, an eight-volume
work that, according to H. Mumford Jones, "was, until de Tocque-
ville, the best French book on the United States" (Jones, p. 151). As
a true representative of the Enlightenment, Liancourt's curiosity extended to everything: politics, constitutions, judiciary organization,
army, agriculture, population, industry, statistics, public welfare, cus-
toms, education. In January, 1796, he was elected to the American
Philosophical Society. On March 4, 1797, he attended the proclamation of John Adams and Thomas Jefferson as, respectively, president
and vice-president of the Republic. As described in his book, Liancourt visited the Pennsylvania Hospital (where, as early 1756, the
first group of mentally ill had been admitted), Dr. Benjamin Rush, and
hospitals and dispensaries in New York. Over and above agriculture
and health, Jefferson and Liancourt also shared an interest in education: In 1786 Liancourt had opened on his estate the *Ecole de Liancourt*, where one hundred orphans and children of military personnel
were taught the various mechanical arts. After his return to France,
he devoted himself to a number of philanthropic endeavors, in particular, the introduction of technical courses at *Les Ecoles d'Arts et
Métiers* (Dreyfus).

Among the letters of Jefferson quoted above there is one to Thomas
Cooper (1759–1839), an Englishman who had studied anatomy, law,
and chemistry in London before settling in Pennsylvania in 1793,
where he later became a state judge. He eventually spent the last
twenty-five years of his life teaching chemistry, first at Dickinson
College, then at the University of Pennsylvania, and finally at South
Carolina College, where he served as president from 1821 to 1834.
During his youth Cooper had come under the influence of French
physiology and had sojourned to France; later, while in South Carolina, he renewed his interest in French matters.

It has been said that Priestley—the great British-born chemist and
theologian who eventually settled in Pennsylvania—represented English materialism, while Cooper represented French materialism (Anderson and Fish). In line with French sensationalism, Cooper taught
and wrote in various tracts that mental phenomena consisted of sen-

sations and ideas and were dependent on physiological processes, affected by diseases, accidents, or sleep.

Less known is the fact that Cooper served on the Board of State Hospitals for the Insane in Columbia, South Carolina, which was originally approved by the General Assembly in 1821 but did not open until 1828 (Hurd). That his interest in the mentally ill was more than casual is proven by his translation into English of Broussais' *De L'irritation et de la folie* (1828) (Broussais, 1831). Francois Broussais (1772–1838) had become known for his fight against the prevailing medical doctrines. More significant, however, was his book on insanity, which, as Ackerknecht recently put it, "was essentially a courageous reaffirmation of Cabanis' ideas on the 'Rapports du physique et du moral'" (Ackerknecht, p. 66). In the introduction to the volume, Broussais stated that "the true medical observation . . . cannot take place except with the intervention of the senses . . . , the abstract scientific ideas cultivated by the spirit come from the senses. . . . Cabanis had gone a step further from the external senses, inasmuch as he recognized the powerful influence of the viscera on thinking . . . and it was advisable to correct Locke's system, but only with Cabanis' approach" (Broussais, 1828).

. Thus, a direct line ties Cabanis to Broussais and perhaps also to Jefferson and Cooper. Judging by the above-mentioned correspondence, Jefferson was apparently aware of Cooper's plan to translate Cabanis. Was he also aware of the moral treatment carried on in France and England and eventually in this country? During the period 1790 to 1800, a decade crucial for the history of the world, psychiatry emerged as a new field and was identified in France with Pinel and in England with William Tuke. Jefferson may have met Pinel at the salon of Mme Helvétius and he may have heard of his reforms at Bicétre and Salpêtrière, his treatise, and his disciples; he may have heard of the treatment used by the Quakers at the Retreat in York, England, and later used in this country in the earliest private mental hospitals.

Jefferson also must have been familiar with Benjamin Rush and his work on behalf of the mentally ill. Jefferson and Rush had met as early as June 15, 1775, at the appointment of General Washington as Commander-in-Chief of the American armies; they had both signed the *Declaration of Independence* the following year; and Rush, not unlike Jefferson, had at times taken such a strong antifederalist and francophile stance as to be called a "French Democrat." Following extended conversations with Rush on the subject of religion, Jefferson sent him, in 1803, a "Syllabus of an Estimate of the Merit of the Doctrines of Jesus, Composed with Those of Others." What unified their thinking was their staunch conviction that happiness, the ultimate goal of man, could be achieved only in a society stable, ordered and stimulating, as typified by the new republic (D'Elia; Weyant).

From all the above it is clear that the connection between the Idéologues and Jefferson may have been closer than had previously been assumed. Many questions, however, must remain unanswered because of the lack of pertinent sources. As Chinard (1925) put it: "It will not be possible to obtain a full picture [of Jefferson's relationship with the American philosophers] until the correspondence between Jefferson and Priestley, Thomas Cooper, Benjamin Rush, Du Pont de Nemours, the Abbot Correa and many others will be finally published."

Cabanis and Jefferson—A Comparison

Toward the conclusion of his study on Jefferson and the Idéologues, Chinard (1925, p. 227) stated: "Among the three [Stewart, Cabanis, and Destutt de Tracy] he [Jefferson] does not see any contradiction. Placing themselves at different viewpoints, they have successfully carried on the most thorough possible research on the means of knowledge. But, of these three philosophers, it is especially Cabanis who catches his attention, because it is in him that he finds a method which most closely resembles that of natural history." Today, fifty years later, this statement by the doyen of the studies on Jefferson and the French culture is still valid. In fact, over and above intellectual affinities, it is possible to uncover other similarities between these two men.

First of all, they both came from an agricultural background and from a small town. Cabanis' father, though a lawyer by training, never practiced law; instead, he devoted himself to the improvement of agriculture by importing and transplanting all sorts of fruits. Probably as a result of this early influence, Cabanis remained attached to country life as long as he lived. Jefferson's father, aside from being a political man, was a surveyor and a civil engineer; thus, the seed of Jefferson's *Notes on the States of Virginia* can be traced directly to his father. He too preferred country life (Binger, 1970). His attempts to improve agriculture by importing all sorts of products are well known.

All that is known of Cabanis' mother is that she died when he was eight. Cabanis was the youngest of three children and the only boy. Rebellious and independent from early childhood on, he was expelled from a religious school. Unable to manage him, his father left him, at the age of fourteen, with his old friend Turgot in Paris, then a high official in the King's service. Cabanis returned to Paris in 1775, at age eighteen, after a long sojourn abroad, and three years later accepted an invitation to remain as a guest of the then fifty-nine-year-old Mme Helvétius at Auteuil. A mother-child relationship developed between them and his need for a mother figure was finally met.

As for Jefferson, he was the first boy of nine children; except for a younger brother, the others were all girls. Though his mother has been described as high-spirited, lively, cheerful, affectionate, humorous, and well educated, he hardly ever mentions her. In his monograph on Jefferson, the psychiatrist Carl Binger (1969, 1970) states that "this can be explained more by a certain shyness in him, and a reserve when speaking of family affairs outside his family, than by any lack of responsiveness or affection. Or perhaps he was too dependent on her and had to assert his manliness by cutting himself off from her." At any rate, the young Jefferson developed a strong attachment to his father. At fourteen, when his father died, Thomas became the oldest male in a family composed of his mother, six sisters, and a baby brother. According to Binger, Jefferson's persistent desire to return home, his passive stance toward his election for president, the maternal role he assumed toward his two daughters after the untimely death of his wife, and finally his aesthetic and artistic interests—from music to architecture—are characteristics of his "feminine" side. This side, not to be equated with weakness or passivity, is to be considered the counterpart of his masculine side, characterized by his aggressive and executive traits and his extraordinary precision of mind.

As regard their personalities, Cabanis has been described by his contemporaries as kind, affectionate, "angelic" (Moravia, 1968), and interested in helping and ministering to the poor. His friends at Auteuil compared him to a Greek thinker. His sensitive disposition is reflected in his many works, all of which are imbued with genuine concern for others and a constant search for improving mankind.

Jefferson, in turn, has been described as cool and reserved, yet as a man of deep sentiment and even warmth. It is well known that he did not like to speak in public; rather, he excelled in writing noted for its depth, knowledge, and style. While Cabanis wrote on broad subjects from a philosophical perspective, Jefferson wrote on more concrete subjects from a common sense perspective. And while Cabanis wrote treatises, Jefferson wrote letters—another "feminine" trait that could be added to those mentioned by Binger.

Both Jefferson and Cabanis received a classical education that influenced their thinking for the rest of their lives. As already mentioned, the seeds of Jefferson's philosophical ideas can be traced to his favorite classics, such as Cicero and Plato, which he read in the original Latin and Greek. Cabanis, too, was familiar with the classics and was fluent both in Latin and Greek. At the age of eighteen, he began to translate Homer's *Iliad* (and the part that he translated was highly praised by Voltaire), a project he resumed in 1807, the last year of his life. Aside from the classics, both men were influenced by the great thinkers of the seventeenth and eighteenth centuries, by Locke and Montesquieu, the Scottish philosophers, the deists, and the materialists.

As a result, they were convinced of the important role the environment—notably education—played in the molding of the young person and of the virtually infinite perfectibility of man. Over and over again an optimistic feeling, consonant with the tenets of the Enlightenment, emanates from their actions and writings—an appealing trait, indeed, though stemming from different sources: Cabanis believed that a new era would emerge from the ruins of the *Ancien Régime,* while Jefferson's enthusiasm was rooted in what he perceived as endless boundaries and opportunities provided by the new nation. Their strong belief in environmental forces and in man's perfectibility was reflected in their concern with education.

Since his early years of colonial public life, Jefferson had made every effort to establish a system of public education, convinced that only through a minimum of education could the democratic principles of the new Republic be made accessible to everyone and be indefinitely preserved (Conant; Honeywell; Lee). Moreover, he spent the last years of his life personally supervising the details of the establishment of the University of Virginia, the first state university in America. He, himself, always studious and inquisitive, was a living example of a man persistently faithful to the educational ideals of the Enlightenment, an example that he tried to pass on to his two daughters.

Cabanis, too, believed in the importance of education, first to achieve and then to maintain and improve the ideals of the French Revolution. Aside from his previously mentioned *Essay on Public Education* (1791), he also reported "On the project of the organization of public schools and, in general, of public education" and wrote a "Report on the organization of the medical schools" both in 1799. He believed that through education, as well as through public welfare and preventive medicine, many evils of society, including mental illness, could be eventually eliminated (Williams, 1953, 1956; Barnard).

Both Cabanis and Jefferson are considered precursors of today's ecological movement. Indeed, it has been said recently that Cabanis' "study of climate as the 'totality of physical circumstances attached to each locality' would be, in modern times, a comprehensive human ecology" (Staum). As for Jefferson, his early book, *Notes on the State of Virginia,* was ecological and makes for refreshing reading today.

Also strikingly similar is the magnitude of their versatility. Cabanis was, in fact, at once a physician, a politician, a literary man, a historian of medicine, and an educator. Jefferson was a pioneer researcher and theorist in the fields of paleontology, ethnology, botany, geography, agriculture, and meterology (Browne; Martin). In addition to being a lawyer, he was a litterateur, an expert in architecture, an educator, and of course, a politician. His interests were so wide and his grasp was so keen that some considered him a genius comparable only to Leonardo.

It is unfortunate that this very versatility has hindered a comprehensive and well-balanced recognition of their contribution to the progress of mankind. Jefferson's importance in political affairs has tended to obscure his significant place in early American science, and Cabanis' dual commitment to medicine and philosophy has militated against a proper appreciation of his contribution to both fields.

Most evident is the difference in their respective roles as seen from the historical perspective: Jefferson's stature continued to increase to the point of almost becoming a symbol of the democratic ideals on which the United States was founded, while Cabanis' name has been relegated to an occasional footnote in scholarly studies and is hardly ever mentioned in publications on the history of psychology and political history. Various factors may have contributed to this difference.

Cabanis lived in an old country in which traditional values were disappearing, soon to be substituted by new values. The ideals of the revolution, first enunciated in 1789 and then reiterated after the end of the Reign of Terror in 1793, were soon to be crushed by Napoleon's imperialism. It was clear that in the new regime set up by Napoleon, the Idéologues, including Cabanis, their most illustrious representative, could only play a minor role.

Cabanis' physiological and philosophical speculations in the framework of the Idéologie were directly opposed to the goals of the newly established French empire. His attempt to relate man's moral traits to bodily traits was viewed as an atheistic stance unacceptable in the new climate of the Concordat with the Catholic Church, signed by Napoleon in 1801.

True, in his *Rapport du physique et du moral,* Cabanis stressed the importance of will over intelligence and, in general, of the intrinsic goal-oriented characteristic of animal life, anticipating Schopenhauer's "will" and Bergson's *élan vital.* Later on, in his *Lettre à M. Fauriel sur les causes premières* (Cabanis, 1806), although he did not refer specifically to God, he considered the vital principle that informs the living body as a substance, a real being; and, going back from effect to cause, he admitted the presence of a primary cause, of a supreme intelligence that regulates the entire world (Joussain; Plongeron).

As for Cabanis' contribution to medicine, despite the following he had among his colleagues, his pioneering insights into mental illness were obscured by Pinel's glory. Regardless of the esteem in which he was held by Broussais and others, his work was considered too philosophical and "vitalistic," and thus disregarded in favor of the histological and biochemical approach to physiology and physiopathology. Only recently, with the advent of dynamic psychology and psychosomatic medicine, has the need for a reassessment of his work and a proper historical evaluation become evident. Certainly, Cabanis' efforts toward public welfare, preventive medicine, and public education were implemented under the Directory (1795–1799) and in the early years of Napoleon's government. But this success was cut short by all sorts of measures—in medicine, welfare, and education—that reflected the totalitarian approach of Napoleon's regime (Vess, 1967, 1975).

In direct contrast to Cabanis' relative obscurity and misrepresentation stands Jefferson's renown and popularity in this country as well as in Europe. But like any brilliant man reaching the peak of a national political career early in life, Jefferson had many enemies. He was accused of being an inveterate opponent to the Constitution, of being immoral, a slave owner, and an atheist. His fight with the Federalists, especially at the time of his election to the presidency in 1801, was extraordinary. Yet, for all this, he had as a young man achieved general recognition as the author of the *Declaration of Independence*, an achievement that opened many doors to him, notably those of the Société d'Auteuil in Paris. The very fact that Jefferson lived in a new country, devoid of centuries-old prejudices, must have contributed to the rapid rise of his glory and to its persistent increase after his death.

Cabanis and Jefferson thus shared many similarities, including their common philosophical orientation: a mixture of methodological ideology, of agnosticism, and of deism that made it possible to assign them to the materialistic as well as the spiritualistic tradition. They also presented many differences, notably between the theoretical speculative, and even utopian thinking of Cabanis and the pragmatic and action-oriented thinking of Jefferson.

As pointed out above, political circumstances restricted the impact of Cabanis' pioneering insights. In that regard, the difference between his fate and that of Jefferson could not be greater. In the spirit of the Bicentennial, therefore, it seems fitting to reassess the reciprocal influence between these two men from the perspective of the ideological movement. Such a reassessment, it is hoped, may also throw new light on the relationship between the old and the new continent, and on the remarkable contribution these two men made to the then emerging field of psychology, as well as the newly established tenents of democracy. Psychology and politics, originating from the same *Zeitgeist*, grew independently for decades and were joined only in recent years by a number of moral, legal, and medical issues. Moreover, problems related to preventive and social medicine as well as to public education, to which both Cabanis and Jefferson addressed themselves, tend to remain complex and unsolved in our day as at their time. A study of the common origins of psychology and democracy may contribute to a solution of these problems.

References

Ackerknecht, E. H., *Médicine at the Paris Hospital, 1794–1848* (Baltimore: Johns Hopkins Press, 1967.

Aldridge, A. O., *Franklin and His French Contemporaries*. (New York: New York University Press, 1957).

Anderson, P. R., and Fish, M. H. (eds.), *Philosophy in America: From the Puritans to James* (New York: Appleton-Century, 1939), p. 249.

Barnard, H. C., *Education and the French Revolution* (Cambridge: Cambridge University Press, 1969).

Benard, R. "Une maison de santé psychiatrique sous la revolution: La maison Belhomme," *Semaine des Hôpitaux, 32:* 3990–4000, 1956.

Binger, C., *Thomas Jefferson: A Well-Tempered Mind* (New York: Norton, 1970.

———, "Conflict in the Life of Thomas Jefferson," *American Journal of Psychiatry, 125:* 1098–1107, 1969.

Blau, J., *Men and Movements in American Philosophy* (Englewood Cliffs, N.J.: Prentice-Hall, 1963).

Boas, G., *French Philosophies of the Romantic Period* (Baltimore: Johns Hopkins Press, 1925), p. 26.

Boyd, J. P. (ed.), *The Papers of Thomas Jefferson* (Princeton: Princeton University Press, 1950), vol. II, 489–491.

Broussais, F. J. V., *On Irritation and Insanity: To Which Are Added Two Tracts on Materialism and an Outline of the Association of Ideas* (Columbia, S.C.: 1831).

———, *De l'irritation et de la folie* (Paris: 1828), introduction.

Browne, C. A., "Thomas Jefferson and the Scientific Trends of His Time," *Chronica Botanica, 8:* 363–426, 1944.

Bruce, W. C., *Benjamin Franklin Self-Revealed* (New York: Putnam's Sons, 1917), chap. VII.

Cabanis, P. J. G., "Lettre à M. F. sur les Causes premières" (1806), in *Oeuvres Philosophiques* (Paris: Presses Universitaires de France, 1956), vol. II, pp. 255–299.

——, "Coup d'oeil sur les revolutions et sur la réforme de la médecine" (1804), in *Oeuvres Philosophiques*, vol. II, p. 77.

——, "Rapports du physique et du moral de l'homme" (1802), in *Oeuvres Philosophiques*, vol. I, pp. 105–631.

——, "Notice sur Benjamin Franklin" (1798–1800?), in *Oeuvres Philosophiques*, vol. II, pp. 341–367.

——, "Rapport sur l'organisation des Ecoles de Médecine" (1799), in *Oeuvres Philosophiques*, vol. II, pp. 405–424.

——, "Sur le projet d'organisation des Ecoles primaires et en géneral sur l'Instruction publique" (1799), in *Oeuvres Philosophiques*, vol. II, pp. 425–450.

——, "Quelques principes et quelques vues sur les secours publics" (1793), in *Oeuvres Philosophiques*, vol. II, pp. 1–64.

——, "Journal de la maladie et de la mort d'Honoré-Gabriel-Victor-Riquetti Mirabeau" (1791), in *Oeuvres Complètes* (Paris: Bossange, 1823), vol. II, pp. 1–78.

——, "Travail sur l'éducation publique" (1791), in *Oeuvres Complètes*, vol. II, pp. 363–581.

——, "Observations sur les hôpitaux" (1790), in *Oeuvres Philosophiques*, vol. I, p. 11.

——, "Du dégré de la certitude de la médecine" (1789), in *Oeuvres Philosophiques*, vol. I, pp. 33–104.

Cailliet, E., *La tradition littéraire des ideologues* (Philadelphia: The American Philosophical Society, 1943).

Canguilhem, G., "Cabanis," in Gillispie, C. C. (ed.), *Dictionary of Scientific Biography* (New York: Scribners, 1971), vol. 3, pp. 1–3.

Cazeneuve, J., "La philosophie de Cabanis," in Cabanis, P. J. G., *Oeuvres Philosophiques* (Paris: Presses Universitaires de France, 1956), vol. I, pp. xxii–xxxviii.

Chabert, P., "Philippe Pinel à Paris (Jusqu'à sa nomination à Bicêtre)," in Blaser, R. U., and Buess, H. (eds.), *Aktuelle Probleme aus der Geschichte der Medizin* (Basel: Karger, 1964), pp. 589–595.

Chinard G., *L'apothéose de Benjamin Franklin* (Paris: La Librairie Orientale et Américaine, 1955), p. 75.

——, "Jefferson among the Philosophers," *Ethics*, 53, 1943.

——, *Jefferson et les idéologues* (Baltimore: The Johns Hopkins Press, 1925).

Colonna d'Istria, F., "Ce que la médecine expérimentale doit à la philosophies: Pinel," *Revue de Métaphysique et de Morale*, 12. 186–210, 1904.

Conant, J. B., *Thomas Jefferson and the Development of American Public Education* (Berkeley: University of California Press, 1962).

Condillac, E. B., "Logic" (1792), in *Oeuvres Philosophiques* (Paris: Presses Universitaires de France, 1947), vol. II, p. 376.

————, *An Essay on the Origin of Human Knowledge* (1756) (New York: AMS Press, 1974).

————, *Treatise on the Sensations* (1754) (Los Angeles: University of Southern California, 1930).

Curti, M., "Psychological Theories in American Thought," in Wiener, P. P. (ed.), *Dictionary of the History of Ideas* (New York: Scribner's Sons, 1973), vol. IV, p. 22.

Dain, N., *Disordered Minds: The First Century of Eastern State Hospital in Williamsburg, Virginia, 1766–1866* (Charlottesville, Va.: The University Press of Virginia, 1971), p. 9.

D'Elia, D. J., "Benjamin Rush, David Hartley, and the Revolutionary Use of Psychology," *Proceedings of the American Philosophical Society, 114:* 109–118, 1970.

Destutt de Tracy, A. L. C., *A Treatise on Political Economy* (Georgetown: Milligan, 1817; (repr. in Dorsey, J. M., *Psychology of Political Science,* Detroit: Center for Health Education, 1973).

————, *Commentary and Review of Montesquieu's Spirit of Laws,* Eng. tr. by T. Jefferson (Philadelphia: Duane, 1811).

Dreyfus, F., *Un philantrope d'autrefois: Larochefoucauld—Liancourt* (Paris: Plon, 1903).

Echeverria, D., *Mirage in the West: A History of the French Image of American Society to 1815* (Princeton: Princeton University Press, 1957; repr., New York: Octagon, 1966).

Fayet, J., *La révolution française et la science* (Paris: Rivière, 1960).

Foucault, M., *The Birth of the Clinic: An Archaeology of Medical Perception* (New York: Random House, 1973).

————, *Madness and Civilization: A History of Insanity in the Age of Reason* (New York: Pantheon, 1965; abridged ed. of *Histoire de la Folio,* Paris: Plon, 1961).

Genil-Perrin, G., "La psiquiatrie dans l'oeuvre de Cabanis," *Revue de Psychiatrie, 14:* 398–418, 1920.

Gillispie, G. C., (a) "Science in the French revolution," *Behavioral Science, 4:* 67–73, 1959.

————, (b) "The Encyclopedie and the Jacobin Philosophy of Science," in Clagett, M. (ed.), *Critical Problems in the History of Science* (Madison: University of Wisconsin Press, 1959).

Gouhier, H., "Cabanis," in Dumesnil, R., and Bonnet-Roy, F. (eds.), *Les Médecins Célèbres* (Paris: Mazenod, 1947), pp. 134–137.

Grange, K. M., "Pinel and Eighteenth-Century Psychiatry," *Bulletin of the History of Medicine, 35:* 442–453, 1961.

Guillois, A., *Le salon de Madame Helvétius: Cabanis et les Idéologues* (Paris: Alcan, 1891; repr. New York: Burt Kranklin, 1971).

Gusdorf, G., *Introduction aux sciences humaines* (Paris: Les Belles Lettres, 1960), p. 393.

Hindle, B., The Pursuit of Science in Revolutionary America, 1735–1789 (Chapel Hill: University of North Carolina Press, 1956).

Honeywell, R. J., The Educational Work of Thomas Jefferson (Cambridge: Harvard University Press, 1931; repr., New York: Russell & Russell, 1964).

Hurd, H. M. (ed.), The Institutional Care of the Insane in the United States and Canada (Baltimore: Johns Hopkins Press, 1916), vol. III, p. 594 (repr. New York: Arno Press, 1973).

Jefferson, T., Notes on the State of Virginia (1861) (New York: Harper, 1964), p. 146.

Jetter, D., "Frankreichs Bemühen um bessere Hospitäler," Sudhoofs Archiv für Geschichte der Medizin, 49: 147–169, 1965.

Jones, H. M., America and French Culture, 1750–1848 (Chapel Hill, N.C.: University of North Carolina Press, 1927).

Joussain, A., "La spiritualité de Cabanis," Archives de Philosophie, 21: 386–409, 1958.

King, L. S., The Medical World of the Eighteenth Century (Chicago: University of Chicago Press, 1958).

Knight, I. F., The Geometric Spirit: The Abbé de Condillac and the French Enlightenment (New Haven: Yale University Press, 1968).

Koch, A., The Philosophy of Thomas Jefferson (New York: Columbia University Press, 1944; repr., Gloucester, Mass.: P. Smith, 1957), p. 57.

Larochefoucauld-Liancourt, F., Voyage dans les Etats Unis d'Amérique fait en 1795, 1796 et 1797 (Paris: Dupont, 1799, 8 vols.; Eng. tr., London: Phillips, 1799, 4 vols.).

Lechler, W. H., Philippe Pinel: Seine Familie, seine Jugend—und Studienjahre, 1745–1778 (München: Medizinische Fakultät, 1959).

Lee, G. (ed.), Crusade against Ignorance: Thomas Jefferson on Education, Classics in Education No. 6, (New York: Teachers College Bureau of Publications, 1961).

Lehec, C., "Biographie," in Cabanis, P. J. G., Oeuvres Philosophiques (Paris: Presses Universitaires de France, 1956), vol. I, pp. v–xxl.

Le Roy, G., La psychologie de Condillac (Paris: Boivin, 1937).

Lipscomb, A. A., The Writings of Thomas Jefferson, Centennial Edition (Washington, D.C.: 1904).

Lovejoy, A. O., "The Theory of Human Nature in the American Constitution and the Method of Counterpoise," in Reflections on Human Nature (Baltimore: Johns Hopkins Press, 1961), chap. 2.

McCloy, S. T., The Humanitarian Movement in Eighteenth-Century France (Lexington: University of Kentucky Press, 1957).

Mackler, B., and Bernstein, E., "Contributions to the History of Psychology: II. Philippe Pinel: The man and his time," Psychological Reports, 19: 703–720, 1966.

Manuel, F., The Prophets of Paris (Cambridge: Cambridge University Press, 1962).

Marset, P., "Veinte publicaciones psiquiátricas de Pinel olvidadas: Contribución al estudio de los orígenes del 'Traité sur le manie,'" *Episteme*, 6: 163–195, 1972.

Martin, E. T., *Thomas Jefferson: Scientist* (New York: Schuman, 1952).

Moravia, S., *Il pensiero degli "Idéologues": Scienza e filosofia in Francia, (1780–1815)* (Firenze: La Nuova Italia, 1974).

———, "Gli 'Idéologues' e l'eta' dei lumi," *Belfagor*, 28: 253–265, 1973.

———, "Philosophie et médecine in France à la fin du XVIIIe siècle," *Studies on Voltaire and the 18th Century*, 89: 1089–1151, 1972.

———, *La scienza dell'uomo nel Settecento*, (Bari: Laterza, 1970).

———, *Il tramonto dell'illuminismo* (Bari: Laterza, 1968).

Norwood, W. F., "Medical Education in the United States before 1900," in O'Malley, C. D. (ed.), *The History of Medical Education* (Berkeley: University of California Press, 1970), p. 474.

Nye, R. B., *The Cultural Life of the New Nation, 1776–1830* (London: Hamilton, 1960).

Picavet, F., *Les idéologues* (Paris: Alcan, 1891; repr., Hildesheim: Olms, 1972; New York: Arno Press, 1974).

Pinel, P., "Introduction," *Traité médico-philosophique sur l'aliénation mentale ou la manie* (Paris: Richard, 1801; Eng. tr. in Zilboorg, G., *A History of Medical Psychology*, New York: Norton, 1941, pp. 329–341).

———, "Recherches et observations sur le traitement moral des aliénés," *Mémoires de la Société Médicale d'Emulation*, 2: 215–255, 1799.

———, *Nosographie philosophique ou la méthode de l'analyse appliqué à la médecine* (Paris: Brosson, 1798).

Plongeron, B., "Nature, metaphysique et histoire chez les Idéologues," *Dix-huitième Siècle*, 5: 375–412, 1973.

Poyer, G., "Les origines de la psycho-physiologie: Cabanis," *Journal de Psychologie Normale et Pathologique*, 7: 115–132, 1910.

———, *Cabanis* (Paris: Michaud, n.d.).

Richmond, P. A., The Hôtel-Dieu of Paris on the Eve of the Revolution," *Journal of the History of Medicine and Allied Sciences*, 16: 335–353, 1961.

Riese, W., *The Legacy of Philippe Pinel* (New York: Springer, 1969).

———, "La méthode analytique de Condillac et ses rapports avec l'oeuvre de Philippe Pinel," *Revue Philosophique*, 321–336, 1968.

———, "Le raisonnement expérimental dans l'oeuvre de Pinel," *Evolution Psychiatrique*, 31: 407–413, 1966.

Riley, I. W., *American Philosophy: The Early Schools* (New York: Dodd, Mead, 1907), p. 17.

Roger J., *Les sciences de la vie dans la pensée française du XVIII siècle*, second ed. (Paris: Colin, 1971).

Rosen, G., "Hospitals, Medical Care and Social Policy in the French Revolution," *Bulletin of the History of Medicine*, 30: 124–149, 1956.

———, "Political Order and Human Health in Jeffersonian Thought," *Bulletin of the History of Medicine*, 26: 32–44, 1952.

————, "The Philosophy of Ideology and the Emergence of Modern Medicine in France," *Bulletin of the History of Medicine, 20:* 328–339, 1946.

Rosengarten, J. G., The Early French Members of the American Philosophical Society," *Proceedings of the American Philosophical Society, 44:* 87–93, 1907.

Rutland, R. A., and Rachal, W. M. E. (eds.), *The Papers of James Madison* (Chicago: University of Chicago Press, 1973), vol. 8, Introduction.

Schneider, H. W., *History of American Philosophy* (New York: Columbia University Press, 1946).

Semelaigne, R., (a) "J. Colombier," in *Les Pioneers de la psychiatrie française avant et après Pinel* (Paris: Baillière, 1930), vol. I, pp. 84–87.

————, (b) "J. R. Tenon," in *Les Pionners de la psychiatrie française avant et après Pinel* (Paris: Baillière, 1930), vol. I, pp. 63–66.

————, *Aliénistes et Philantropes: Les Pinel et les Tuke* (Paris: Steinheil, 1912).

————, *Philippe Pinel et son oeuvre au point de vue de la médecine mentale* (Paris: Imprimeries Reunies, 1888).

Staum, M. S., "Cabanis and the Science of Man," *Journal of the History of Behavioral Sciences, 10:* 140, 1974.

Stein, J., *The Mind and the Sword* (New York: Twayne, 1961).

Taton, R., "The French Revolution and the Progress of Science," *Centaurus, 3:* 73–89, 1953.

Van Doren, C., *Benjamin Franklin* (New York: Viking, 1938), chap. 22.

Van Duzer, C., *Contribution of the Idéologues to French Revolutionary Thought,* Studies in History and Political Sciences, Series 53, no. 4, (Baltimore: Johns Hopkins Press, 1935).

Vess, D. M., *Medical Revolution in France: 1789–1796* (Gainesville, Fla.: University Press of Florida, 1975).

————, "The Collapse and Revival of Medical Education in France: "A Consequence of Revolution and War, 1789-1795," *History of Education Quarterly, 7:* 71–92, 1967.

Weiner, D. B., "Le droit de l'homme à la santé: Une belle idée devant l'Assemblée Constituante: 1790–1791," *Clio Medica, 5:* 209–223, 1970.

Weyant, R. G., "Helvétius and Jefferson: Studies of Human Nature and Government in the Eighteenth Century," *Journal of the History of the Behavioral Science, 9:* 29–41, 1973.

Williams, L. P., "Science, Education, and Napoleon I, *ISIS, 47:* 361–382, 1956.

————, "Science, Education, and the French Revolution," *ISIS, 44:* 311–330, 1953.

Woods E. A. and Carlson E. T. The psychiatry of Ph. Pinel, *Bulletin of the History of Medicine, 35:* 14–28, 1961.

H. F. Ellenberger

12

Carl Gustav Jung:
His Historical Setting

No teachings can be fully understood without an adequate knowledge of their author's life and personality. Let us, therefore, briefly review the historical, ethnic, cultural and family setting of Carl Gustav Jung. We have to deal with three kinds of data: (1) the "current version," which may be true or not, but is endowed with a psychological reality of its own, (2) the objective findings, and (3) the unknown history.

The current version is told everywhere and seldom questioned. Much of it is based upon family tradition and hearsay; when comparing this version with objective findings, one is amazed at the number of discrepancies. Relatives, friends, colleagues—all of them in good faith—make inaccurate, incomplete, and sometimes fictitious statements. Not infrequently, a joke is taken at face value and will later be included in the biography as historical fact.

Objective research, based on documents and the testimony of reliable persons, fills many gaps, corrects inaccuracies, and dispels legends. Unfortunately, most of the time objective findings cover only part of the story. Much of the accepted version can be neither confirmed nor disproved, so that gaps are left in our knowledge. Thus, these valuable fragments of truth can produce only an incomplete picture.

This essay was originally presented at the meeting of the American Psychiatric Association in Anaheim, California, May 7, 1975, and is reprinted with the author's permission.

The unknown history is that part of the biography which we do not know and often do not even suspect. Much of it has just been forgotten. But there are also events that have been deliberately concealed by an individual or his family. The veil of oblivion drops rapidly upon a man after his death, inflicting on him, as it were a second death.

Jung's personality reflected to some extent the spirit of his home town, Basel. At the border of three countries (Switzerland, Germany, and France), Basel is an almost unique example of a city-state, with its own government, assemblies, ministerial departments, and administrations. In the days of Jung's youth, Basel was small enough for all its citizens to know each other.

During the Renaissance, Basel was a center of European humanism, the town of Erasmus, Vesalius, Paracelsus, Platter, and the painter Holbein. Then came a period of decay, but the nineteenth century brought a cultural revival: Basel produced a number of original and creative personalities, such as Bachofen and Jacob Burckhardt. Among the men instrumental in the city's cultural revival was Jung's grandfather, Carl Gustav Jung the Elder (1794–1864).

Jung the Elder was a remarkable personality about whose life it is often difficult to disentangle truth from legend. He was entrusted in 1822 with the professorship for anatomy, surgery, and obstetrics in the Medical School in Basel. He gradually restored the school, which had fallen into a pitiful state of decay, to its previous fame, was elected rector of the university, wrote a few scientific treatises, and became a sought-after consulting physician.

His first wife died prematurely, leaving him with three children. According to family legend, his second marriage occurred in a rather unusual way. He went to the Mayor of Basel, and asked him for the hand of his daughter, Sophie Frey. The mayor refused, whereupon Carl Gustav went directly to a tavern and asked the waitress there if she would marry him. She immediately accepted. To be sure, this story could have begun as one of the sarcastic witticisms customary in Basel. The second wife died three years later and left two more children. This time, he did marry the mayor's daughter, who also eventually left him a widower after having presented him with eight children.

Jung the Elder, by most accounts, was a man of irresistible charm, kindhearted, tactful, and humorous. However, one of his sons has depicted him as a despotic father, and the problems he had with several of his children darkened his later years. A touch of secretiveness in his nature led him to write two plays on political topics under pen names. And then there was the mystery surrounding his birth.

According to rumor, Jung the Elder, was an illegitimate son of

Goethe. In August, 1793, Goethe sojourned for some time in Mann-heim, where he could have met Sophie Ziegler, the future wife of Franz Ignatius Jung. However, there is no proof of this, and while Jung, the psychiatrist, is often mentioned as the originator of this rumor, he later came to deny it, sometimes indignantly, sometimes smilingly. But, strangely enough, the birthdate of the elder Jung is disputed. We agree with Johannes Tenzler that two dates would be necessary to give a definitive clue: the exact birthdate of Jung the Elder, and the date of the marriage of Franz Ignatius Jung and Sophie Ziegler.

The semilegendary figure of the grandfather had a powerful im-pact upon his grandson, even though the latter was born eleven years after his grandfather's death. Although his first name was spelt "Karl" in city records, the psychiatrist adopted the antiquated spelling of "Carl" as if to identify himself with his illustrious grandfather.

Notable are the modern psychiatric insights that abound in the Elder's writings and activities. With his definition of mental illness borrowed from Ideler—"the loss of the power of directing oneself ac-cording to one's own determination"—he believed in the efficacy of psychic therapy. When it was decided to create an asylum in Basel, for instance, he took a firm stand in favor of a hospital where patients would be treated instead of receiving merely custodial care. This prin-ciple was no matter of course at that time. In addition, he founded an institution for mentally retarded children. In an article on nostalgia, he claimed that it is not a mental disease as such, but can become one if the patient keeps his suffering a secret. This emphasis upon the deleterious effect of secretiveness anticipates his grandson's future teaching of the pathogenic secret.

The psychiatric principles of Jung the Elder are thus an inter-mediate link between the Romantic psychiatry of Ideler and the later dynamic psychiatries of Freud, Bleuler, and Jung.

As to Jung's grandmother on his father's side, Sophie Jung-Frey, nothing is known, except that she was the mayor's daughter and that she died at the age of forty-three. Samuel Preiswerk (1799–1871), Jung's grandfather on his mother's side, belonged to an old Basler patrician family, and was a protestant minister and professor of Hebraic studies. He became the antistes, or president, of the Com-pany of Pastors in Basel. With his first wife he had one child who also became a pastor and hebraist; with his second wife he had twelve children, of whom the youngest was Emilie, the psychiatrist's mother.

If family stories are to be believed, Samuel Preiswerk had con-versations with spirits, especially with the spirit of his first wife, for whom he had a special armchair in his study and who, he felt, visited him once a week, to the sorrow of his second wife. When he composed his sermons, his daughter Emilie stood behind him, so that the spirits could not read over his shoulder. He promoted the teaching of Hebrew on the grounds that it was the language spoken in heaven.

It is not legend, however, that Samuel Preiswerk militated in favor of the Jews' return to Palestine. His Zionism was based on the conviction that prophecies concerning the Jews would soon be fulfilled. He founded a journal, *Das Morgenland,* the first issue of which began with a manifesto: Israel is the only people whose name was given by God Himself, and the promise made to Abraham, Moses, and David has never been cancelled. *Das Morgenland* went so far as to blame the Jews for a supposed lack of interest in their promised land.

As similar views were held among many Swiss Protestant fundamentalists and pietists, it was not by chance that the First International Zionist Congress took place in Basel in 1897. At the time of the congress, Jung was a twenty-two-year-old medical student, and its events, as we shall see, were reflected in the mediumistic experiments he conducted with his young cousin.

About Jung's maternal grandmother, Augusta Faber, little is known. The story goes that at eighteen she fell into a cataleptic state and was believed to be dead; the coffin was brought in, but at the last moment her mother brought her back to life with a hot iron. She was said, to possess second sight and to have transmitted it to her daughter Emilie, who in turn transmitted something of it to Carl Gustav.

The following generation, that of Jung's parents, was devoid of any romantic features. Each of them was the thirteenth child in an impoverished family.

Jung's father, Paul Achilles Jung (1842–1896), displayed a strong interest in classical and Oriental languages, as shown by his dissertation, which dealt with a commentary on Solomon's Song of Songs by Jephet Ben Eli, a Jewish scholar who lived in Mesopotamia in the tenth century A.D. The commentary was written in Arabic, but with Hebrew letters. Paul Jung transcribed it into Arabic script, translated parts of it into German, and concluded with his own brief remarks. It was an honorable piece of research and the usual opening to a career as an orientalist. But Paul Jung took up theology instead, and spent the rest of his life as a modest country minister. He married Emilie Preiswerk, and then became a pastor in Kesswil (where Carl Gustav was born), later in Laufen, and finally in Klein-Hüningen, near Basel.

According to most accounts, he was a good man, well liked and respected by his parishioners. I once met an old woman who had known him when she was a child. She remembered how once she had to stay at home because of illness, when all her friends had gone on an excursion, and pastor Jung brought her a little gift to cheer her up. According to another account, his colleagues considered him somewhat dull and boring.

In his *Memories*, Jung complained that his father dispersed himself in futile activities and that his personality development had stopped with his student years. Jung also had doubts about his father's faith. However, it would seem that his negative attitude was not free from a certain envy: He never reached his father's mastery of Latin (as reflected in one of his dreams), for instance.

The life and personality of Jung's mother, Emilie Preiswerk (1848–1923), are also far from well known. The same old woman who told me about the pastor's kindness described his wife as fat, ugly, authoritarian, and haughty. But there are other statements. Jung, for one, said that she had two personalities, which may just mean that she was a woman of changing moods.

Jung grew up in the Protestant's presbytery, a setting that has been called "one of the germinal cells of German culture." The Klein-Hüningen presbytery had been the country house of a rich Basler patrician family, and it is conceivable that spending his childhood in such a mansion later influenced Jung to build the splendid house in Küssnacht.

One of Jung's aphorisms was that "nothing is more important in the destiny of a man than the life his parents have not lived." This undoubtedly applied to Jung himself. He compensated in his own life for the lack of ambition he had sensed in his father's life. His wide erudiction in the history of religions was more like that of a theologian than a physician. It is as if he had taken over these studies at the very point at which his father had given them up.

When he asked his father embarrassing questions, he was told that what mattered was to have faith. Jung himself, however, adhered to the principle of "I cannot believe in what I do not know, and in what I know I do not need to believe." In another example, Jung said that as a young boy he wondered about the mystery of the Trinity and waited eagerly for the explanation his father would give in catechism class, but when they came to it, his father merely said that he himself did not understand it. It is significant that, much later, Jung published a paper with the title "A Psychological Approach to the Dogma of the Trinity. Still more significant is a letter a Protestant minister wrote him expressing doubts about his vocation, exactly the problem Jung assumed his father had had. In his reply, Jung discouraged the pastor from leaving the ministry, explaining that doubts are not contradictory to Christianity, but rather reflect a deepening of certain experiences on which the Christian faith is based.

Jung was not quite four when the family moved to Klein-Hüningen. He first went to the village school, where his father taught him Latin. At age eleven, he went to the *Gymnasium* (secondary school) in Basel. Here, as in Klein-Hüningen, he felt himself set apart from the other pupils, most of whom belonged to well-to-do families. This might account for his later, somewhat megalomaniacal, daydreams, in which he identified his "second personality" with a prominent character of the eighteenth century.

At the *Gymnasium*, Jung received a classical humanistic education. He attended catechism courses taught by his father; he also took a passionate interest in the philosophies of Schopenhauer and Nietzsche, in current psychological research on hypnotism and multiple personalities, and in spiritism.

Jung was twenty when he registered at the Basel University medical school. His father was already sick, and died a few months later. As a result he, his mother, and his sister had to leave the presbytery and rely upon the help of relatives. These were years marked by poverty, but also by intensive studying and a keen interest in the unknown realm of the mind.

Jung had only one sibling—his sister Gertrud, who was nine years younger—but he had numerous relatives. He was on good terms with the younger children of his uncle Rudolf, particularly with his cousins Luise and Helene. These two belonged from the start to the circle in which he performed the spiritistic experiments that provided the data for his medical dissertation.

Until now these facts were known only from Jung's dissertation, from a 1925 seminar, and from his autobiography. In my book, *The Discovery of the Unconscious*, I have identified the medium. The medium's niece Stefanie Zumstein, recently revealed abundant details about these experiments; her account, however, differs greatly from Jung's version. As she explains it, Jung changed the chronology of the experiments, concealed important facts, and modified the order of the mediumistic manifestations. According to Jung, the experiments started in July, 1899, and ended in the fall of 1900. Stefanie Zumstein maintains that they began as early as June, 1895, and went on, with several interruptions, until September, 1899. Jung also said that he joined an already organized group, but Mrs. Zumstein contends that he was the initiator.

The first three séances took place in June and July, 1895, in the presbytery of Klein-Hüningen, with five participants: Carl (the only man): his mother, Emilie; his cousins, Luise and Helene Preiswerk;

and Helene's intimate friend, Emmy Zinsstag. Nobody's father was told about it. Carl was twenty years old; Luise, twenty-one; and Helene, thirteen and a half. From the start, Helene showed remarkable mediumistic abilities. She fell into trances and the voice of grandfather Preiswerk spoke from the other world through her about certain painful events in the Preiswerk family. In the second séance, grandfather Carl Gustav Jung the Elder, was supposedly present with grandfather Preiswerk, but he did not speak.

After an interruption of several years—Jung's father and Helene's father had died—the séances started up again. Several other Preiswerk girls joined the group, and Helene became more and more the focus of attention.

Following the First International Zionist Congress, the spirit of grandfather Samuel Preiswerk appeared again and entrusted Helene with the mission of bringing the Jews to Palestine and converting them to the Christian faith. From then on, the séances took place more frequently, though at irregular intervals. In the summer and fall of 1898, the medium began to reveal some of the secrets of the spiritual world: she spoke about the planet Mars with its canals, vegetation, and inhabitants, and about her successive reincarnations, beginning with having been a woman loved by King David, and terminating with having been a young woman seduced by Goethe, which made her Jung's great-grandmother.

At this point, Jung invited several fellow students to a séance, which disturbed the medium's capabilities; but in order not to disappoint her beloved cousin, she simulated her mediumistic condition. When this became obvious, Jung discontinued the experiments.

In August, 1899, the séances were resumed, but Helene's revelations met considerable resistance within the family. A period of violent family disputes followed, and Helene's mediumism came to an abrupt stop. According to Mrs. Zumstein, the séances continued, however; the medium was now Jung's sister Gertrude, but her brother was no longer interested.

Stefanie Zumstein insists that behind these spiritistic experiments, Jung was carrying on a romance with his two cousins. Luise, six years younger than Carl, had for some time been living in the presbytery, and Helene came often to visit her sister. For a while, Carl was in love with Luise, but Helene was deeply in love with Carl, and had boundless admiration for him. However, she kept her love to herself. Her mediumistic manifestations, probably genuine enough at first, gradually became a desperate means of attracting Jung's attention and gratifying his expectations.

Soon after the end of these experiments, Jung passed his final medical examinations, completed his military service, and became a psychiatric resident at the Burghölzli mental hospital, in Zürich. He chose as his M.D. dissertation topic the mediumistic experiments with his cousin, which appeared in 1902 under the title *On the Psychology and Pathology of so-called Occult Phenomena.*

Jung then took a leave of absence from Burghölzli to spend the 1902–1903 winter semester in Paris and study with Janet. This period is not mentioned in his autobiography, and until recently belonged to the "unknown history."

Stefanie Zumstein found three letters written by Jung during his stay in Paris. Helene and Valerie Preiswerk were studying dressmaking and lived in Versailles with their friend, Emmy Zinsstag. Jung lived in Paris and sometimes visited his cousins. In two of the letters, he invited Helene to spend an evening with him at the theater. He seems to have been very fond of her, but by then he was engaged to Emma Rauschenbach, the daughter of a wealthy Schaffhousen industrialist; he married her on February 14, 1903.

Meanwhile, his dissertation had been published and had become known in Basel. Although he had used pseudonyms and altered the chronology, the identities of the characters were soon recognized. Some of his descriptions were rather unflattering and many Preiswerk relatives were deeply hurt. In those days considerable stress was put on heredity, and the whole maternal side of the family appeared to be tainted with insanity. Rumors circulated that the younger Preiswerk daughters could not find husbands because of Jung's dissertation and that Helene had died from a broken heart. Actually, she died from tuberculosis at the age of thirty.

Whatever criticism could be made of Jung's dissertation, one major point is clear. He implied that Helene's psychic growth was impeded by psychological and social obstacles and that her mediumistic utterances were a means resorted to by the unconscious to overcome these obstacles. We recognize here the origin of Jung's theory of individuation, the most crucial concept in his psychological system and therapy.

Part IV

Mind-Brain Relation in Historical and Philosophical Perspective

Four of the authors in this section discuss aspects of the unconscious, and several others discuss the future: Baruk treats moral and social responsibility; Reinhold, survival of the human species; Ey, Syz, and Lhermitte, man's sound or disturbed functioning and the purpose or mode of relief. Gooddy's essay is concerned with cerebral and biological adaptation to the fast-moving, swiftly changing, four-dimensional world in whose terms man is progressively thinking. The essay shows that history is the expert's harbinger of tomorrow's thought and science.

All the authors in this section have been alive to influence or inspiration from the past. Not unexpectedly, then, each one arrives at his conclusions as the result of an historicocritical evaluation of thought and discovery in his field. Reviewing critically 150 years of predominantly French anatomo-clinical research, Baruk concludes that the problem of the neuroses cannot be attacked without previously studying the problems of the nervous system and the relations of its disorders to psychological disturbances. He regrets that Freud's psychogenetic approach led him to declare an excess of control to be pathogenetic. It is rather the loss of control in organic cases that causes the release of behavioral excesses. In nonorganic cases, it is the repression of man's inherent and powerful conscience that causes the unleashing of hatred and, in turn, the conflicts and formidable shocks of human history.

In a letter mentioned by Baruk, Doryon alerts Freud to the view that his theory deifies the uninspirational and demoniacal forces; it does not lead, as in Freud's Hebraic tradition, to their diffusion. However, Baruck acknowledges that Freud abandoned psychophysical mechanisms for the human personality in its infinite dimensions.

Syz, on the contrary, sees the peril arise from within man's conscious mind. In common with Burrow and others, he states that there could be no war without symbolic function that presumes the framework of ideologies. He recognizes, however, that issues are not clearcut. The conflict in man does not reside within man's rational mind alone and his privilege to make choices. It is also one of biocentric versus the logocentric attitude.

According to Reinhold, man is at the mercy of his ancient, unconscious, resilient, genetically determined urge to increase his species, whereas his biologically recent and highly developed conscious mind realizes that uncontrolled growth of population menaces the species with extinction. The gap in communication between the conscious and unconscious mind is due to a dual system of language—one of qualification, the other of quantification. The latter can be applied to the body, not the mind. This duality has isolated man from his origins and natural environment. In an increasing number of ways, the extinction of life (including his own) becomes more probable as quantifying language enchants him with its magic, his quantifying ingenuity succeeds, and his conceptual thinking remains devoted to physical and chemical phenomena. For individuals, as well as society, Reinhold suggests psychotherapeutical techniques to resolve the conflict between conscious and unconscious mind.

Syz has studied Burrow's origination of group therapy and the results of Syz's study have Burrow's philobiological and philoanalytical basis. In Syz's view as in Reinhold's, language began the conflict between early and recent aspects of human development by alienating man from himself and his environment. Reinhold considers the danger to be in the species attributes of man, whereas Syz, with Rousseauistic perspective, sees the danger in the development of man's symbolic capacity—in particular, speech. It alienates him from the immediacy of experience.

Syz's studies have the additional importance of having been acquired by participation in group sessions where there was no distinction between the sick and the well. Minute self-observations of psychosomatic reactions were made, and the resultant data indicated that the psychophysiological processes involved are characteristic of human nature generally and not specific to particular personality organization or cultural patterns. The literature Syz discusses is voluminous and of great interest.

The essay by Lhermitte and Signoret concerns language itself. They are pioneers in the most recent approach to the interpretation of aphasia—an approach based on neuropsychology and linguistics. Although these disciplines derive from a variety of sources, there are precursory indications of the new approach in Walther Riese's writings—namely, in his elicitation of the limits of neuroanatomical research. He implied that future studies should be concerned with a dimension identical to that of the studied object. Ey also arrives at this thought, though on different paths. Both he and Riese elaborate on the reasons why the anatomical substratum is silent to our inquiry in principle or under specific circumstances. The contribution of Lhermitte and Signoret consists in their disregarding the silenced and unrevealing space for the study of the surviving function, which is the affected speech itself. By choosing the science of linguistics, they confine themselves to the dimension of language.

Lhermitte conceives of speech as detached from thought. He bases this concept on an analysis of the literature and on his own experiments with Signoret and others. Like Henry Head, Lhermitte believes that, by the use of signs, speech mediates between conception and oral expression or, in Ombredanne's formulation, the explicit elaboration of thought. The sign replaces the image, and signification (meaning) replaces representation. He defines aphasia as a defect of utilization of the rules permitting the encoding and decoding of a verbal message.

For forty years, Ey has been captivated by the theories of Hughlings Jackson, an English country physician. Jackson's views on the function and dysfunction of brain-mind relationships form the fundamental body of modern neurology. Ey analyzes Jackson's theories, and as a result, delineates the territory and defines the meaning of mental illness as opposed to neurological symptomatology. Since only the latter had been Jackson's concern, Ey's is an original contribution. For both men the unconscious is the automatism set free by the dissolution of the higher levels of brain function. Dissolution reverses the path of evolution, and since the highest levels of mental function are the last in evolution, they are the first to fall prey to dissolution. According to Ey, they must be regarded not only as instruments of consciousness but as instruments effecting the integration of the nervous organization as a whole—that is, including themselves. Loss of the highest levels, therefore, results in diffused symptoms that defy localization. Such symptoms are the reason why purely psychogenic theories of mental disease or emotional aberration could develop. The highest levels being those of global integration, their dissolution causes global or uniform disintegration, which concerns the field of psychiatry; the dissolution at subordinate levels causes partial or instrumental disintegration, which concerns the field of neurology. The mental symptoms observed in defects of the higher levels—symptoms such as illusions and hallucinations—seem to be positive, but they are not. They are not the direct effect of the lesion. "Disease does not evolve the new; it produces only negative mental symptoms resulting from the dissolution. The apparently positive symptoms are the outcome of activities untouched by any pathological process and are the exaltation of certain faculties that the well-preserved layers of function keep under control."

The articles of Reinhold and Gooddy reflect two opposite views of life. Whereas Reinhold is concerned with mankind's possible extinction, Gooddy forecasts a new dimension of human development. However, having been close collaborators for years, they developed a simple test that has had far-reaching consequences. Their test confirms Gooddy's hypothesis that a specialization of potentialities exists in the symmetrical hemispherical brain structures: On the one side is the instrumentality of language, and on the other, space-time skills. Man is developing an economy of anatomical structures subserving these functions.

Gooddy associates this brain development with man's escape from Darwinian evolution to a four-dimensional concept of space-time. Forms of specialization of nervous performance tend, mainly without consciousness, toward the need for obviating millions of years of gradualness. This idea implies completely new rates of space-time awareness for the human race. Gooddy affirms that the separation of space and time is passing from us. New notions of time, memory, and age will establish themselves in us as we extend our range of speed and space. Gooddy suggests that such an anthropological development might well be a worthy subject of interest for the neurological clinician.

Henri Baruk

13

Modern Neuropsychiatry and Freudian Psychoanalysis: A Historical Study

One cannot attack the problem of neuroses without studying the relations between disorders of the nervous system and psychological disturbances.

It should be remembered that for a very long time psychological disturbances were thought to be independent of somatic factors and ascribable solely to psychical factors. This theory of the separation of body and mind was still dominant when it was brought into question again in 1822 by the discovery of general paralysis at Charenton. We know that Bayle at first differentiated this new affliction on the basis that patients suffering from it displayed mental disorders at the same time as motor disorders, revealing an incomplete paralysis. Moreover, Bayle, after anatomoclinical investigations, attributed both the psychical and motor symptoms to a single cause, chronic arachnitis, in other words, to a special lesion of the meninges and the brain, described later as meningoencephalitis and finally as general paralysis.

In attributing the psychological impairment as well as the somatic impairment and the paralyses to the same anatomical cerebral cause, Bayle knew that he opened the way for a new unicistic doctrine of mental diseases.

But at the time, this unicist conception was strongly opposed, notably by Baillarger, who defended the dualist notion that only the motor disorder depended upon the meninges and the brain, while the mental disorders constituted a mental disease, paralytic insanity, arising solely from psychological causes. More than a century of investigation, notably the work of Calmeil at Charenton and Griesinger in Germany, was needed to confirm Bayle's doctrine.

But the great founders of modern psychiatry, Pinel and Esquirol, had not committed themselves in that direction. The method Pinel valued above everything was clinical observation and description of symptoms inspired by scientific methods. This is why he gave an unforgettable description of mania. Esquirol at Charenton followed the same course, presenting a memorable description of most of the principal mental syndromes and examining puerperal psychoses from the etiological standpoint. Yet they took little heed of the hypothesis presented by Bayle. Bayle was supported instead by his master, Roger Collard, physician-in-chief of Charenton, and was besides a follower of Laënnec, the creator of the anatomoclinical method in medicine.

It was by virtue of this anatomoclinical method that neurology was created at the end of the nineteenth century by Charcot. There then came into being a new field of medicine, that of physical disorders associated with localized lesions of the brain or spinal cord. Neurology was founded upon direct links between pathological symptoms and anatomical lesions, whence the extensive development of cerebral anatomy and anatomophysiology, making possible the exact tracing of the centers and the pathways of transmission. The very model of these investigations was pyramidal hemiplegia associated with anatomical impairment of the pyramidal tracts either at the level of the anterior ascending tract or of the internal capsule, or lower down at the level of the protuberance or the bulb. Disorders were explained exactly by anatomical interruptions without the intervention of other factors. After the pyramidal tract, the syndromes of impairment of the extrapyramidal tracts were studied with Parkinson's disease or the striatal syndromes, and the same thing was done for disturbances of the sensory functions and of speech. Thus, a veritable cerebral geography was established.

However, clinical experience was already demonstrating that certain patients had analogous disorders without anatomical cerebral lesions. There were descriptions of psychical hemiplegias, of mutism simulating aphasia—all of which were results of a different disease, described by Sydenham under the name of "the great simulator," that is, hysteria. The simulator included the epileptic attack, but without complete loss of consciousness, without cyanosis, etc.

Thus began the chapter of the neuroses. To give an example: We saw a patient complaining of hemianesthesia, the complete absence of sensation of one half of his body. When we touched the skin on this half of the body, he declared he felt nothing. Then we made this absurd request: "Tell me each time that you do not feel anything." At each touch of the finger on this supposedly insensitive region, he replied with absolute precision: "I don't feel it," thus demonstrating that his disorder was only psychical, a sort of belief in his hemianesthesia, or what Bernheim (at Nancy) then described as suggestion, and what Babinski later called unconscious simulation.

So it was that Freud, arriving from Vienna to complete a training course in Paris at the Salpêtrière in Charcot's service, was confronted with the problem of hysteria. Imbued with the doctrine of localizations, Charcot explained hysteria as a functional disorder of the same centers the anatomical lesions of which produce organic neurological disorders. For example, hemiplegia, through injury to the internal capsule brings about paralysis of one half of the body. So, thought Charcot, a functional disorder of this same zone (leaving the nerve centers intact) would cause psychical or hysterical hemiplegia. According to this conception, the anatomical impairment of the speech center would produce aphasia, while if only functionally disturbed, it would produce a merely psychical disorder of speech, mutism.

This so-called organodynamic conception of Charcot's was thus narrowly focused upon cerebral localizations. It was brought into question again by the substantial work of Babinski.* He discovered, in fact, a series of objective signs indicative of injury to different localizations, for example, disturbances of the plantar reflex (Babinski's sign) in pyramidal disorders, and special signs of asynergia in the cerebellar syndrome.

These signs are absent in hysterical hemiplegia and in all other hysterical syndromes. Moreover, in hysterical hemiplegia, the attitude of the muscles is coordinated as in a voluntary attitude, whereas in organic hemiplegia there occur dissociations in muscular attitudes that cannot be produced at will and are inimitable.

Lastly, as final proof, Babinski showed that hysterical accidents (notably hemiplegia) were totally and immediately curable by persuasion, that is, by psychological action, while organic accidents did not react at all to such therapeutic action. Babinski distinguished sharply between organic neurological manifestations and manifestations similar in appearance, but psychical and of hysterical nature. Furthermore, Freud knew Babinski. He was perfectly conversant with all these facts and had come into contact with Bernheim, who had discovered the influence of suggestion.

Freud began his studies on hysteria with Breuer. After abandoning the use of hypnosis, he began to resort to an analysis of dreams or of abortive acts to assemble the thoughts beyond conscious volition, which, in his opinion, were the sources of neurosis.

---

*Claude and Ey tried in vain to reestablish it, and we have related the conflict with which we were faced on this point to our teacher, Claude, and our colleague, Ey.

The notion and the term neurosis appeared belatedly in the history of psychiatry. All the very important work of Pinel and Esquirol and of their numerous nineteenth-century successors is concerned only with serious mental disorders expressed in delusion, excitation or depression, or weakening of the intellectual faculties. In contrast, Freud was interested only in the new concept of psychological disturbances hidden behind purely physical disorders in subjects retaining normal lucidity and behavior.

Another form of neurosis had been described in the memorable works of Pierre Janet on obsessions and psychasthenia. Here, also, it is a matter of lucid subjects of apparently normal actions who complain of an invasion of their consciousness by an idea foreign to their thoughts. Here the disturbance is not (as in hysteria) a neurological disorder but an incoercible, annoying thought of which the subject is fully aware, which he criticizes, and against which he struggles. This distinguishes him radically from the subject with a behavior disorder, the isolated and subjective psychological disturbance that was designated a psychoneurosis or obsession.

This whole territory of the neuroses was to constitute the field of Freud's work and the domain of psychoanalysis.

To understand Freud's position in this field, previous work in French psychopathology should be reviewed. Any observer can readily notice that what characterizes neurotic disorder is lack of control: The subject in an attack of hysteria cannot master the emotions that cause him to writhe; the subject in a state of obsession cannot suppress the alien ideas that sweep into his consciousness and terrify him.

During the course of French psychopathology, this weakening of control was attributed to the nervous system's causing a predominance of automatism over controlled activity. So it is that Baillarger (who extended this conception to the psychoses), writes that such disorders are caused by "the involuntary exercise of the mental faculties." Later, Pierre Janet, returning the same thesis, describes them as due to a special torpidity that would prevent consciousness from controlling the lower activities. De Clerambault later develops this thesis again, but for him mental automatism, concretized in hallucinations often athematic or impersonal and giving rise to delusion, comes from cerebral irritation by the sequelae of infection or intoxication. Later, in our work on experimental catatonia, we identified the nature of the torpidity pointed out by Pierre Janet, showing that it was of toxic origin, and we were able to bring to light a series of poisons of volition, certain ones of which have their source either in the intestine (Vincent's neurotropic toxin from the intestinal colon bacillus) or in bile (with Camus). Also demonstrated was the toxic origin of that torpidity of the will akin to sleep that we designated as "cataleptic sleep" and the psychophysiology of which we studied. This new current led back to the conceptions of Moreau de Tours, who, as far back as the mid-nineteenth century, had shown the analogy between the dream and insanity, had related psychopathic disorders to a wakeful dream, and had indicated the kinship of delusion to sleep when sleep invades waking life, forming a mixture of dream and reality.

Such are the stages of French developments concerning disorders in the mechanisms of thought. All these works are based on psychophysiology, and thus depend more or less on scientific facts.

Freud's position is diametrically opposed. Abandoning the objective and general point of view of psychophysiology, Freud transfers the problem to the subjective and individual plane. For him it is no longer a question of psychophysiological relaxing of control, but, on the contrary, a question of an excess of inhibition related to social conditions. In order to conform to conventions and social obligations (represented by the Freudian superego), the subject has suppressed affects, intense desires— libidinous for the most part and often inadmissible—that, thrown back into the unconscious, emerge regularly in dreams or in abortive acts, and that afterwards form the content of neurosis. Freud's aim is not, therefore, to reinforce censorship, but rather to neutralize it in order to let the repressed emotional charges rise to the surface of consciousness and, thereby, to defuse them.

The problem thus posed by Freud is a subjective and individual problem. It is a matter not of impairment in psychophysiological mechanisms that control thought, but of a personal life story. It is a matter, moreover, of a finalist interpretation of neurosis, suppressed desires acting and imprinting certain attitudes that seem incomprehensible according to logic. That is the great Freudian revolution. It consists in restoring to importance the desires, instincts, and dynamogenic tendencies that were misunderstood or reduced to factitious elements in rationalist conceptions of man.

Man thus no longer consists solely of rational and logical consciousness; behind this consciousness there exists an immense hidden domain from which come inspiration and unexpected impulses that shock and can overpower the human being.

But why should Freud have seen fit to shrink this immense unconscious sea of man to sexual desire alone and to unavowable desires for pleasure in conflict with social requirements? Here is apparent the strong influence upon Freud of certain Teutonic ideas that glorify nature and instinct and evade moral and social imperatives prevalent in Wagnerian ideology, sometimes brutally affirmed in the cult of force, sometimes even (as with the famous character expert Klages) in the intoxication of destruction. Invaluable elucidation on this subject will be found in the correspondence exchanged between Israel Doryon and Freud.[1] Doryon does not fail to reply to Freud that the God of Abraham, Isaac, and Jacob maintains himself above the nature that he created and does not identify himself with it. One may remember that God humanizes nature by opposing to the reign of force that of *Tsedek*, the very source of humanity. To act righteously, to seek truth, to see oneself in one's neighbor's place, such is the foundation of the Torah as opposed to myths of force, fate, or predestination by the stars.

The ardor for justice of the Hebrew prophets, which protests strongly against oppression of the weak or the underprivileged, which sustains the weary or discouraged and raises them up again (without, however, transforming this liberation into a revolution), which upholds the innocent, which defends truth against the lure of false truths —this ardor, which, ever since the prayer of Hannah, the Psalms of David, and the Prophets, has uplifted the world—this ardor, astonishingly enough, remained extraneous to Freud, although he was Jewish by birth.

This ardor for justice which comes from heaven (*min hashamaim*) inspired the Prophets and created the phenomenon of *N'vouah*, with its inspirations and voices as well as the phenomenon of the *She'hinah* (Divine Presence), which we have studied in a recent work.[2] The unconscious of the Prophets and of men of faith was filled with this altruistic and ardent inspiration, which gave them the meaning of the march of humanity towards Messianism and universal peace.

As for Freud's unconscious, it finds its inspiration in selfish desires, in sensual and lewd impulses, in covetousness and sometimes hatred of one's fellow being, in debased lives of a crude nature knowing neither good nor evil, nor social and moral obligations, nor the interdicts that they entail. Any God of this unconscious belongs to the *shedim* (demons), to the factors of force and violence individualized in the term *Azazel* (evoking, according to Ramban, the outrages and aggressiveness of Esau). All these forces incontestably exist in the depths of the human soul, and it was certainly naïve to wish to repress them and shut them up in a sealed unconscious. The Hebraic tradition has been well aware of them, but it attempts not simply to restrain them, but above all to defuse them under the enlightenment of Divine Power.

Freud, on the contrary, deifies them and ascribes to them an exclusive and predominant role in man. Without realizing that he is referring to some of the same forces so stressed in the Hebraic tradition (practices of accusation, *hasatan mekatreg*), he incessantly accuses: He accuses victims of complicity with their aggressors, a theory afterwards developed by Mendelsohn. This theory results in the removal of culpability from aggressors and the justification of their action. Therein lies the danger of Mendelsohn's victimology.

In this perspective, Freud attacks the well-known verse of Moses (Leviticus, XIX): "Thou shalt love thy neighbor as thyself," which he considers a "*credo quia absurdum*." He goes on to attribute the grief of mourning to the unconscious and suppressed wish to kill the departed loved one. Likewise, he glorifies the basest forms of instinct and considers that they should be brought out in the open.

Thus, Freud's work, while noteworthy for the restitution of human personality in some of its infinite dimensions, operates in such a way that, instead of restoring this personality to complete integrity, it reduces it to its inferior components, divorces its carnal impulses from social factors, and thus deprives the human being of the powerful inner judgment of moral conscious, which we have studied anew and which, when repressed, gives rise to terrifying hatreds and lays the foundation for personal conflicts and the formidable convulsions of human history.

Finally, psychoanalysis has assumed the form of an exclusive dogma that claims to explain everything. The fact that it has had the merit of renewing interest in the subjective life and the individual's life story, however, should not blot out or fuzz over the role of disorders of the nervous system or the very important achievements of neuropsychiatry from the nineteenth century through the beginning of the twentieth.

References

1. Freud et le Monothéisme Hébreu. L'Homme Moise, par Israel Doryon. Préface de Prof. H. Baruk, Traduit de l'hébreu par H. Baruk et Weisengrun. (Paris: Editions Zikarone, 1972).
2. H. Baruk: *La Névouah et le Prophétisme à l'Etat Normal et Pathologique dans l'Histoire des Individus et des Peuples.* Annales, Medicopsychologiques Tm II h⁰ 5 Dec. 1973, pp. 593–624.

Margaret Reinhold

14

Darwinian Evolution
of Certain Aspects of Mind

*So we beat on, boats against the current, borne back cease-
lessly into the past.*

—F. Scott Fitzgerald, *The Great Gatsby*

In spite of centuries of debate by philosophers and scientists, there is
no satisfactory definition of "mind," yet mind has a practical significance for physicians. Physicians believe pragmatically in psychosomatic illness, disturbances of body function coexisting with emotional or mental stress. It has also been observed that certain disturbances of mind occur in conjunction with disease of or injury to body.
Certain aspects of mind are thus regarded by physicians as interfunc-
tioning with body.

The hypothesis that mind has evolved in the Darwinian sense,
together with body, depends on the assumption that mind/body relationship does exist, and takes into account the concepts of "consciousness" and "the unconscious."

The unconscious mind of man has been studied since the beginning of this century, notably by psychoanalytical methods that, however, tend to relate to modern man in Western societies. Despite the
limitations of such theories, it is now generally accepted that unconscious motivations may influence human behavior.

An attempt will be made here to see man in the context of evolution: a small, lonely animal, newly emerged from the three thousand
million years of life that have preceded him. Although he has much
in common with his ancestors and also with many other species at
present in the world, contemporary man has forgotten his origin. The

events of the last few thousand years and, in particular, the last hundred years, have contributed to his increasing isolation from his environment and from his predecessors.

At present, man appears to be firmly set on the road to extinction as a species. Yet, since the body of man incorporates genes that might be as old as life itself, it is possible that there are aspects of mind that are also of very ancient origin. Thus, the mutating genes that caused the infinitesimally slow changes in body also influenced mind. It is the aim of this essay to present man's dilemma as related to the evolution of mind.

THE IMPORTANCE OF ACTIVITY OF BODY AND MIND AS RELATED TO EVOLUTION

Throughout the life of an organism, both body and mind function in a state of continuing activity. Activity of body consists, of course, of physical and biochemical activities of an ordered, sequential nature, by means of which body cells maintain a constant equilibrium essential for the preservation of life.

During life, mind is also in a state of unending activity of an ordered nature. Those aspects of mind that coexist with functions of body demand action from mind—that is, the maintenance of the state of consciousness, the maintenance of the unconscious, the performance required for perceiving sensations, for going to sleep (and staying asleep), for conceptual thinking, remembering, forgetting, learning, and so on. All these performances demand complex and continuing activity of mind, and if mind ceases to maintain such activity, disturbances of both body and mind occur (Reinhold, 1951, 1954, 1955; Gooddy & Reinhold, 1952, 1953).

On a practical basis, confusion in the description and analysis of functions of mind and body may be avoided by using language strictly appropriate to the activities of each of these two aspects of man. Human language consists of two systems. One system describes quantity, including symbols that are able to define quantity with extreme precision. The language of physics and biochemistry belongs to this system. This language has also provided man with the key to understanding one of the most important aspects of being—the physical structure and biochemical activities of genes.

The second system deals with quality, and describes aspects of being that are not amenable to quantitative analysis, for example: mind, consciousness, the unconscious, sensations, and mood.

While body, or cell, activity is described in the language of quantification, mind and behavior may not be so described. In other words, since mind and body interfunction, there are two kinds of happenings occurring simultaneously, but the happenings occur in a parallel manner in time. At present, we have no language system that could make the relationship between events in body and events in mind more understandable.

To demonstrate the hypothesis that certain aspects of mind have evolved in the Darwinian sense, two aspects will be analyzed in detail: perception and instinctive behavior.

PERCEPTION

Perception is here defined as a property of mind, the conscious experience of sensations (as seeing, hearing, tasting; feeling pain, heat, cold, fatigue, hunger, thirst, and so on). Such stimuli occur as successive events in time and are ceaselessly in operation. The processes inside the body may be described in terms of physical and biochemical activities. In the mind of man, in common with certain other animals, there also occur activities such as integration, selection, suppression, contrasting, and associating. Such activities occur in the unconscious mind, where an important activity is the attribution of spatial characteristics to perceptual experience. Sensations are perceived as occurring within or on the surface of the body, outside the body, above or below the body near or far from the body, larger or smaller than the body, but always in relation to the body. Perceptual experience depends on impulses that pass from every part of the skin, from every organ, from every joint, from every muscle, up and down and around the nerves, the spinal cord, and the brain (Gooddy). Thus, a man or an animal has a precise mental knowledge of his position in space, the size and posture of his body and limbs, and the position of every part of his body in relation to gravity (Schilder). Just as the impulses traveling around the nervous system are in constant activity, so the mental image of the body is constantly changing, and mental activity is required to keep the body image in equilibrium. The perceptual image of the body is so precise that such infinitely delicate sensations as a fine hair on the tongue or the twitch of a few muscle fibers may be located on or in the body. The attribution of a location in space to sensation is an activity of mind.

As body changed and evolved, as the upright posture evolved, as hand structure and handedness evolved, as eyes and ears, nose and tongue evolved, so also did the body image change and evolve. Therefore, perceptual experiencing, which is inextricably welded to the body image, has also evolved.

The activities of genes are probably related to the potential for an activity of mind or body, rather than to the activity itself. Learning an aspect of mind, must play an important role in the achievement of activities of both body and mind of any organism (Thorpe).

EVOLUTION OF INSTINCTS

Instinctive behavior is a response to stimuli originating from the environment or within or upon the surface of an organism's body. While such responses occur in living organisms that cannot be said to possess mind in the medical sense, these responses may be regarded as aspects of mind in its most primitive, rudimentary form.

Certain instinctive responses may be highly complex and linked to other instincts. For example, aggression may be linked to preservation of territorial rights. Many instincts are linked to the most compulsively motivating instinct of all, the instinct to survive. Instinctive behavior patterns may be accompanied by affect in those animals potentially able to experience it—affect being a mood or emotional state such as fear, unhappiness, or pleasure. The motivations for instinctive responses belong to unconscious mind, but the affect that may accompany instinctive responses is experienced in conscious mind.

When an organism has the potential for a variety of instinctive responses, possibilities exist for considerable flexibility in terms of response to stimuli.

Certain animals, including man, have the potential for instinctive:

Sexual behavior patterns or drives to procreate
Aggressive behavior patterns
Submissive behavior patterns
Ritualistic behavior patterns, both among members of the same species and between one species and another
Grouping behavior
Behavior creating and sustaining family systems
Isolation
Migration
Hibernation
Bonding
Communication by signals or language
Obsessionalism
Preference for heights
Preference for enclosed spaces
Preference for open spaces
Establishment and preservation of territorial rights

Establishment of pecking orders, and many other patterns of behavior

Much behavior belonging to instinctive patterns of response may be learned by the younger generation from its parents, only the potential for the instinctive pattern being inherited. Since it has been clearly demonstrated by geneticists and animal behaviorists that the potential for instinctive behavior is inherited, it must be said that instinctive behavior evolves (Lorenz, Tinbergen).

In man, unconscious (instinctive) reactions may be examined by conscious mind. A certain degree of conscious control of instinctive reaction then becomes possible.

Discussion

As certain aspects of mind evolve in the Darwinian sense, the implications of this evolution are of importance with regard to the survival of man as a species.

Evolving mind made a contribution to the survival of species as did evolving body. In early forms of life, the contribution of evolving mind to the survival of a species may have been of lesser importance than evolving body, but the more complex mind became, the greater its contribution to the success (or failure) of a species' survival. Those aspects of mind that are understandably of value to survival include not only instinctive reactions, but the affect accompanying and intensifying such reactions. Examples of powerfully motivating affect belonging to mind are hunger, thirst, fear, and anger.

With the gradual evolution of consciousness and conceptual thinking, evolution of body became less important. Survival no longer depended solely upon mutation of genes, for mind could promote survival by making increasing use of its potentials. Mind was and is self-generating. It is capable of establishing behavior patterns by conceptual thinking, and such patterns may be passed on to the next generation.

Animals in whom consciousness has evolved are able to aid consciously at survival. Consciousness permits animals to choose actions—the choice being limited by the animal's capabilities and by the actions available—provided the options open to the animal are recognized by conscious mind. It is thus possible for animals such as man, with a highly evolved potential for consciousness and conceptual thinking, to aim at survival in immediate contingencies. Man is also able to plan behavior aimed at survival in the future, for he is able to predict contingencies. It must again be emphasized, however, that conscious mind, a relatively recently evolved aspect of mind, cannot efficiently control behavior patterns motivated by the unconscious, which remains the most potent and compulsive aspect of mind.

Unconscious mind operates in terms of ancient instincts—a vast quantity of compelling, inherited strategies for survival, evolved over an immense period of time.

Many animals have highly evolved minds and a high capacity for consciousness, and affect efficient ways of receiving and using sensory information and powerful armaments of instinctive reactions. Perhaps the most important ability of modern man has been his capacity to devise complicated systems of language, particularly the language of qualification. Since qualifying language can be applied only to activities of body and cannot be applied to mind, modern man, entranced with the success of his quantifying ingenuity, has tended, in the last century, to devote his conceptual thinking to physical and chemical phenomena.

In addition to remarkable benefits, technological developments have also created great problems, such as overpopulation, energy shortages, and pollution. Many species of animals and birds have been eliminated, and man himself is threatened as a species. The main cause of danger has not been man's abilities of consciousness and conceptual thinking, nor the language that quantifies; it is that man has continued to function largely in terms of unconscious mind while simultaneously using conscious conceptual thinking to plan survival. Man is thus at the mercy of unconscious, genetically determined urges to increase his species, while at the same time he recognizes, on a conscious level, that an uncontrolled increase in population means man's eventual decline as a species.

CONCLUSION

Mind is a phenomenon accepted pragmatically in the practice of medicine. The language of quantification, which cannot be applied to mind, has so captivated man that insufficient attention has been paid to mind.

All psychotherapeutic theory and practice accept the concepts of conscious and unconscious mind. The aim of psychotherapy is to bring unconscious motives for behavior into consciousness, after which, in theory, the individual in treatment becomes able to make conscious constructive choices regarding his actions. It is suggested that, if it is not already too late techniques might be applied to both individuals and societies to resolve the conflicts between conscious and unconscious mind.

REFERENCES

Freud, S., Works of Sigmund Freud (London: Hogarth Press & The Institute of Psychoanalysis).

Gooddy, W., "The Circulation of the Nerve Impulse," Lancet, 451, 1957.

Gooddy, W., and Reinhold, M., "Some aspects of human orientation in space I." Brain, 75: 472, 1952.

———, "Some aspects of human orientation in space II." Brain, 76: 337, 1953.

Jung, C. G., The Collected Works of C. G. Jung (London: Routledge and Kegan Paul).

Lorenz, K., "Über die Bildung des Instinktbegriffes," Naturwiss, 25: 298, 1937.

———, "The Comparative Method in Studying Innate Behaviour Patterns," Symp. Soc. Exp. Biol. 4 Animal Behaviour, Cambridge 221, 1950.

———, "The Role of Aggression in Group Formation," Trans. of 4th Conference on Group Processes (New York: Josiah Macy Jr. Foundation, 1960).

———, Das Sogenannte Böse, zur Naturgeschichte der Aggression (Dr. G. Borotha—Schoeler Verlag, 1963).

Reinhold, M., "Some clinical aspects of human cortical function," Brain, 74: 339, 1951.

———, "An Analysis of Agnosia," Neurology, 4, No. 2, p. 128, 1954.

———, "Certain disturbances of attention associated with organic cerebral disease, Brain, 78: 417, 1955.

Schilder, P., The image and appearance of the human body. Psyche Monographs No. 4 (London: Kegan Paul Trench Trubner & Co., 1935).

Thorpe, W. H., Learning and Instinct in Animals (London: Methuen, 1963).

Tinbergen, N., An Objectivistic Study of the Innate Behaviour of Animals. Biblioth. biotheor. 1, 39, 1942.

———, The Study of Instinct (Oxford University Press: 1951).

———, Social Behaviour in Animals (London: Methuen, 1953).

———, "Some Aspects of Ethology, the Biological Study of Animal Behaviour," Advan. Sci. 12: 17, 1955.

———, Proc. Roy. Soc. (London: Ser. B) 182: 385, 1973.

———, B. B. C. 2 Television. "The World About Us" programs. (Windrose & Dumont—Time. BBC Hamburg, 1974).

Hans Syz

15

Value Problems in Psychotherapy against the Background of Trigant Burrow's Group Analysis[1]

In attempting to find reliable criteria for appraising values that reside in the participants in psychotherapeutic situations and in the therapeutic process itself, we are confronted with a somewhat bewildering complexity of variable factors, with a diversity of individual needs and ways of life that are interwoven with sociocultural value systems. If we should agree that our therapeutic efforts aim at advancing individual growth and self-actualization in the setting of constructive relatedness, we have made a general statement that permits different interpretations. These interpretations depend in part upon the therapist's personal and cultural background, upon his preconceived image

---

1. An abbreviated version of this essay appeared in the *International Journal of Group Psychotherapy*, vol. 11, April 1961, pp. 143–165. It was first delivered at the Sixteenth Annual Conference (1959) of the American Group Psychotherapy Association before a panel on "Methodological Problems Involved in Evaluating Values in Group Psychotherapy." Problems of value have long been of interest to me, especially as they relate to my association with the pioneer studies in group dynamics introduced by Trigant Burrow in the early 1920s. Though a forerunner of various group psychotherapeutic movements, Burrow's group analysis was based upon somewhat different premises, and it offers an altered perspective for evaluating the therapeutic process generally.

In 1963, Dr. Riese wrote a perceptive historical review of Burrow's conceptions in which he related them to earlier scholars. The following essay does not attempt any such broad survey, but rather recounts the development of Burrow's researches from the position of a participant. I have let the main themes stand as they were written seventeen years ago and have merely added a few footnotes in order to update certain aspects. I would formulate some of the issues differently today, but the essential problems presented in the essay are still relevant.

of man, and upon his ideas regarding maturity, mental health, and the therapeutic process. These and other determinants embody interrelational attitudes and evaluations of which we are hardly aware and which may either further or impede the therapeutic endeavor. An especially complicating factor lies in the circumstance that we observe and experience behavior and values only as totalities in which dynamic processes from different sources are merged and in which it is difficult or impossible to discriminate between the different components (constructive and neurotic-defensive; conscious, preconscious, and unconscious).

On the basis of my participation in Trigant Burrow's group-analytic investigations, I would like to suggest that these problems of value orientation are in part related to a socially systematized impediment, in ourselves as well as in our patients, that subtly restricts observation, concepts, and evaluations. We found this impediment to be connected with complications that arose in the use of image-symbol functions within the processes of human awareness, of individuation, and of interchange, and with the resulting deflection of attention upon the self-image. I shall outline the methods we used in observing and working with this adaptive malfunction. But before taking up these problems of perspective from the background of Burrow's phylo-biological researches, a few general considerations are called for.

VALUES, SCIENTIFIC METHOD, AND MENTAL HEALTH

The following methodological problems appear especially pertinent with regard to value assessment: First, we may ask what we really mean by the terms value and evaluation. Second, we may consider the relation of values and evaluation to science, that is, whether values can be investigated and appraised at all in a scientific manner, what scientific methods have been employed so far in the approach to values, whether values can be changed by scientific investigation, and how far they may influence scientific pursuits. Third, we may review special difficulties that are met, conceptually and operationally, in psychotherapeutic settings, and perhaps in educational pursuits generally, in which we aim to establish a reliable frame of reference for value judgments.

Value and Evaluation

We find that various investigators writing on value theory (Lepley, 1949), or what is called axiology, emphasize not only that values and evaluations are inherent features of human action, but also that they

are influenced by knowledge, by advancing interpretations of the objects, actions, and experiences to which they refer. Ralph Barton Perry
(1954) defined value in terms of interest; values have a dynamic connotation; they relate to goals, desires, attitudes, and motivations. As
Charles Morris (1956) put it, values refer "to the actual direction of
preferential behavior toward one kind of object rather than another."
Or again, in Kluckhohn's (1954) formulation: "A value is a conception,
explicit or implicit, distinctive of an individual or a group, of the
desirable which influences the selection from available modes, means
and ends of action." These definitions emphasize that affective (desirable), cognitive (conceptual), and conative (selective), elements
are essential to the notion of value, and they include the individual's
relation to group and culture. Evidently, any evaluation presupposes
a specific value orientation of the appraiser.

Scientific Procedure

With regard to scientific procedure, the question has been asked
whether it can be of service in value problems. In discussing the contributions to a symposium entitled "Values in Action," sponsored by
the Wenner-Gren Foundation for Anthropological Research, Conrad
Arensberg (1958) concluded: "Morals and values are unarguable, absolute. . . . For scientists to debate morality as scientists, rather than as
citizens or believers, is not only an invasion of the rights of citizens, it is
an implied arrogation to scientists of expert status and expert authority
above that of other citizens." In an editorial in the issue of *Human
Organization* in which the report on this symposium appeared, it was
agreed that values cannot be scientifically determined, but it was suggested that the values of scientists, while not publicly debated with an
effort to convert the other fellow to one's own point of view, might
be publicly presented and discussed. It was added that "anyone involved in an effort to apply his research findings is necessarily involved
in value problems."

A number of investigators, for instance Emerson (1954), Gerard
(1942), Goldstein (1947), Herrick (1926), von Monakow (1927),
Riese (1938), and Sinnott (1955), have discussed what they consider
the biological foundations of ethical values. They proposed that basic
prerequisites for ethical values can be understood in terms of biological
organization, although they recognized that forms of choice and responsibility exist on the human-cultural level that are not found in
infrahuman organisms.

The close relation of science to values was emphasized by Conant
(1953), who pointed out that the activities of scientists are shot
through with value judgments. He agrees with the trend in twentieth-

century science to consider scientific theory as a policy, a fruitful guide to action. Science is a dynamic enterprise in which a series of interconnected concepts and conceptual schemes, arising from experiment and observation, leads to further experiments and observations. Human conduct, value judgments, common sense, and scientific concepts closely interpenetrate, and scientific discovery has to fit the times. Or, as Schrödinger (1952) put it, all science is value oriented, and in the last analysis, "is an integrating part of our endeavor to answer the one great philosophical question which embraces all others—who are we?" There is a question in how far science can lead to an increasing cognitive approximation of the ultimate structure of the world. Bridgman (1950) even suggested that "the structure of nature may be such that our processes of thought do not correspond to it sufficiently to permit us to think about it at all"[2]

Not only does the influence of values upon science express itself as a positive directive force, but values may impede scientific activity and progress. We know how such value judgments as scientific dogmas, personal preconceptions, and culturally conditioned ideologies have delayed the acceptance and fruitful development of scientific findings and conceptions. Especially in the behavioral field, they may prevent the investigator or the public from asking the right questions and from establishing an adequate basis for the investigative process. The self-defensive reinforcement of personal value systems may lead to a competitive opposition of theories and to an overemphasis upon unessential distinctions that are not supported by the structure of the material examined.[3]

With regard to the specific application of scientific methods to value problems, we have, for instance, "A Clinical Study of Sentiments" by Murray and Morgan (1945). These investigators reject the idea that science is not concerned with values; they emphasize that

---

2. Such conclusions arising in modern science derived from experimentation are sometimes paralleled or confirmed on levels of experience where the limitations and relativity of perception and conception come directly to awareness. An instance of such awareness, experienced in my youth, is reported in *Vom Sein und vom Sinn* (Syz, 1972).

3. The determining function of coherent traditions in scientific research has been discussed extensively by Thomas S. Kuhn (1962). He points out that "normal science" presupposes accepted models or "paradigms," which include specific types of law, theory, application, and instrumentation. Scientific practice within such frameworks inevitably evokes "crises," which may be resolved by "scientific revolutions." A new gestalt may suddenly appear and with it a new scientific perception and interpretation of the world. The change to another paradigm permits the search for novel facts and theories. A particular set of shared values is important in directing the scientific process.

the psychologist "should eventually be able to provide a foundation for a pragmatic system of values."

Another effort to investigate values was reported by Charles Morris in his *Varieties of Human Value* (1956). He stated that a scientific axiology, or unitary pattern of value theory, may develop "that will be an essential part of the emerging science of man," and that "in influencing our appraisal, [this axiology] may well affect profoundly our preferential behavior itself." Further aspects of the relation of values to science have been taken up by Hartmann, by Margenau, and by Bronowski in *New Knowledge in Human Values*, edited by Maslow (1959).[4]

Summarizing these comments on values and science, we may say that (1) scientific procedure appears to include evaluations as guiding or as inhibiting factors, (2) important aspects of values can be investigated by scientific methods, and (3) scientific investigations and accumulating knowledge or insight may play an important part in changing existing value orientations.

Values in the Psychotherapeutic Setting

With regard to the criteria for appraising values in the psychotherapeutic situation, we may say that these values are related to what we assume to be man's propensity for creative autonomy and socially cohesive functions on the one hand, and to certain impediments, resistances, or obstructions to the basic need for growth and contact with others and the world, on the other hand. Observations made in various forms of psychotherapy demonstrate that increasing knowledge or conceptual clarification is at least one factor that may change the appraisal of values—and the values themselves—that motivate the participants in the therapeutic encounter.

The difficulties involved in establishing a generally valid frame for assessing values in the psychotherapeutic situation are linked in part to differing concepts of mental health and mental illness. Riese's (1953) historical review of the conception of disease discussed the many perspectives from which the phenomena of health and disease have been approached in the various stages of medical doctrine. While there is no line between health and disease, Riese emphasized a concept that, as he pointed out, has its forerunners in early Greek philosophies: the formulation that disease represents a complex organization of vital manifestations that, although characterized by internal

---

4. Value and motivation are closely interconnected. A thorough discussion of theory and research in the field of motivation has been given by Cofer and Appley (1965).

discord, also includes constructive, formative factors. Riese showed that health and disease are not tangible objects but concepts, products of thought, conceived with the purpose of synthesizing—of bringing system and order into—a large range of perceptible phenomena.

In discussing various theories of normality and mental disorder, Redlich (1952) pointed out the shortcomings of statistical, normative, and clinical criteria. He arrived at the conclusion that the various propositions regarding normality contain value statements, that we do not have a knowledge of the essential nature of man adequate to form a universal concept of mental health, and that conceptions of normality are meaningful only in a specific cultural setting and in operational terms. Marvin Opler (1956) also emphasized that the basic emotionality involved in a certain form of adjustment (specific repressions, identifications, sublimations, and defenses) depend to a large extent on the specific ways of life, meanings, and values inherent in a particular family, status group, and culture. We also find that values and behavior patterns characteristic of the psychiatrist's immediate background, as well as of his larger national and cultural group and of the scientific tradition to which he adheres, influence his preference for specific psychiatric theories and therapeutic procedures.

Two important research projects in social psychiatry in which samples of the total population were examined highlight the complexity of the factors with which we are confronted. In the Midtown Manhattan study (Srole et al., 1962) psychiatric and sociological investigations of a 1% sample, selected at random from the 170,000 people living in the Yorkville district of New York, in May 1953, showed that about 25% of the people (not 10%, as is generally suggested) were seriously enough disturbed so that they would benefit from formal treatment. Only about 18.5% were considered free of signs of mental disturbance. The other study (Leighton, 1959–1963), carried out in a rural district of Stirling County, Nova Scotia, corroborated this prevalence of neurotic trends. Leighton pointed out that our knowledge of causative social factors is very inadequate and that our psychiatric facilities cannot cope with the existing mental health problem.

One may ask whether even the relatively few symptom-free individuals may not embody socially systematized dynamics that have pathogenic implications. Another question is, how far does this widespread disposition toward behavioral pathology embody hostile-destructive trends that not only may lead to individual disorders but also may constitute an essential cause of social and international conflict, particularly when they are organized in ideological frames and activated in terms of self-defensive group formations.

In the face of this cultural relativity and of the great diversity of both constructive and noxious factors within the individual and culture,[5] the question arises whether it is at all possible to arrive at common denominators, at a "valuational base or a unified configuration of aspirations in the lives of man" (Edel, 1953), that would permit a comprehensive evaluation and formulation of the dynamics that either favor or impede healthy integrative functions. Basically, the movement *Toward a Unified Theory of Human Behavior* (Grinker, 1956) is in accord with the general trend in science toward relatively simple interpretations of complex data. Thus, we find converging trends in psychopathological schools, attempts to amalgamate Freud, Jung, and Adler, and efforts to integrate psychoanalytic principles with sociocultural dimensions or the existential movement. We begin to understand some of the earlier behavior theories as fragmentary and prematurely hypostatized aspects of a more encompassing conception that has not yet been adequately formulated. This tendency toward unitary, overall conceptions is expressed in the attempts toward transcultural or universalistic definitions of mental health (Jahoda, 1958; Smith, 1950), as well as in certain motivational theories (Allport, 1953; Goldstein, 1947; Whitehorn, 1954).

In discussing the inadequacies of existing concepts of mental health, Thibaut (1943) suggested that Trigant Burrow's phylobiological requirements might permit a coherent and objective formulation of behavioral norms. That is, "no behavior-adaptation within the single individual can be healthy and complete in the absence of a healthy basis of behavior-adjustment within the community as a whole" (Burrow, 1937, p. 414). This shift of emphasis from individual adjustment to a species-wide reorientation, based on careful analysis of inadequate individual and social responses, opens a broadened perspective. The principle of *phylo-organismic integration,* postulated in this connection by Burrow (1930), implies a conceptual and attitudinal readjustment that could provide valid criteria for consistent and comprehensive evaluations.

It is evident, then, that there is a widespread effort to define basic human traits that, while expressed in and modified by culture, have a generic psychobiological background. According to Bidney (1947) and Spiro (1954), the creation and transmission of culture demands a generic human nature or psychobiological structure that is independent of specific conditioning and learning. While there is an endless variety of culturally shaped communicative devices, we find a common structure in man's emotional attitudes and gestural reactions

---

5. For a variety of theories and clinical concepts of mental health, see also Offer and Sabshin (1966).

(Darwin, 1872). Likewise, we may conceive that important aspects of behavior disorder do not vary much in their fundamental structure, in spite of the great variety of individual and cultural expressions. On the basis of such common principles of behavior, a common value orientation may develop.

CONCEPTUAL PREREQUISITES

We have, then, on the one hand, accumulating observations on the great diversity of value orientations, personality formations, and pathological developments that are interrelated with different cultural patterns, and on the other, a growing tendency toward determining basic human needs and values and toward finding common causes and dynamics of behavior disorders. Burrow's group-analytic studies are an important contribution in this search for common characteristics of human nature and its disordered functions. On the basis of specific observational data, a biosocial or phylobiological frame of reference was developed that permitted a more encompassing perspective for value judgments with regard to behavioral health.

In this connection, I should like to emphasize the importance of organismic and configurational principles in the approach to behavior and associated value problems. Terms such as dynamic structure, field, organization, gestalt, figure-ground, functional patterns, and integrative systems express this trend (Syz, 1936). There also is an accent on form in modern physics, expressed, for instance, by Schrödinger (1952), who said: "What is permanent in these ultimate particles [of matter] or small aggregates is their shape and organization. . . . They are, as it were, pure shape, nothing but shape; what turns up again and again in successive observations is this shape, not an individual speck of material."

In the field of living beings, Bertalanffy and Woodger (1933) effectively synthesized available biological data in support of the organismic point of view. Bertalanffy (1950) stressed that living organisms are open systems that not only maintain themselves through interaction with the environment, but also have a compelling tendency to develop increasing complexity and states of higher order. That is, the processes involved go beyond mere homeostasis, with its self-preservative implications; they include growth and differentiation, inherent autonomy, and creative functions. Similarly, Gerard (1958) came to the conclusion that living things show a steady and seemingly irresistible trend toward orderliness and organization. As Riese (1942) put it, integration within the living organism consists of a "mobile hierarchy" of structural and functional patterns. Paul Weiss (1958,

p. 184) stated that in biology we deal with dynamic patterns in which structure derives from function. In a sense, structure is a cross section through a process, and the basic thing is the ordering, formative quality of this process. In the hierarchical order of systems, a relative constancy of phenomena on a "higher" level may occur without corresponding constancy at the "lower" level. While the various levels of phenomena are interrelated and interdependent, novel and unpredictable features may emerge whose characteristics cannot be reduced to the terms of constituent factors; they have to be dealt with by concepts and methods attuned to the specific level of organization. But emphasis on the total configuration does not preclude exact analysis of parts or subsystems, although the part always has to be considered in relation to the total configuration (*ganzheitsgebunden*).

The consistent application of the configurational model allows for complex genetic-causative as well as teleological or goal-directed dynamics, including human purpose. It automatically eliminates mistaken alternatives relating to the mind-body problem or to the controversy between mechanistic and vitalistic interpretations. Further, we may say that the organismic-configurational concept is a prerequisite to an integration of physiological, psychological, and sociocultural factors. This does not necessarily imply the application of an organic theory to society, a position that has been much discussed and criticized (Sapir, 1917; Kroeber, 1917; Goldenweiser, 1917). Rather, we may think in terms of a general system theory that recognizes analogous principles or patterns existing on different organizational levels and in different scientific fields. While manifestations on the sociocultural level may be recognized as distinctive features, we have to take into account the fact that the elaborate symbol and language activity in humans has dynamic forerunners in the sign reactions and communicative devices occurring at infrahuman levels. It is also important to recognize that patterns of neuromuscular activation and their internal perception appear to be significant factors in human emotion, thinking, and social interchange. However, although we consider symbolic-cultural manifestations as aspects of human biology, this does not necessarily imply a reduction of higher level phenomena to terms of lower levels.

With regard to behavior problems, Goldstein's (1939) organismic concept, supported by rich empirical data, has had far-reaching influence. Angyal's (1941) holistic personality theory, which includes social integration, also is of importance. Goldstein's organismic-configurational approach, with its recognition of systems in which part and whole are interdependent, helps us to understand how apparently distant and externally different phenomena may be integral components of a common dynamic structure or may be related to a common denominator. We are thus given a conceptual tool that permits us to understand that what appears to be a localized disturbance may involve the total configuration, and that an adjustment at a pivotal point may bring about significant changes throughout the total pattern. This configurational conception naturally applies also to the socioindividual continuum, to the interactive structure of the individual within the group or phylic setting. In fact, not only may we apply the *concept* of configuration in our thinking, but we may also realize through *experience* that dynamic organization determines all phases of life and behavior.

GROUP ANALYSIS

I took part in the studies of human interaction introduced by Trigant Burrow in the early 1920s. In the course of these studies, an observational technique and a frame of reference were developed that permits a reappraisal of socially sanctioned inadequacies or immaturities in which the observer himself is an interacting participant. Because this research provided an altered perspective for considering problems of value and orientation in psychotherapeutic pursuits, it merits a historical review.

A few words should first be said about certain conceptual innovations Burrow introduced before he took up group work. Though he was a charter member of the American Psychoanalytic Association, he deviated early from Freud's concept that the essential cause of neurotic disorders consists of a conflict between instinctual drives and social prohibitions. Instead, he proposed in his psychoanalytic papers that the conflict derives from the encroachment of the objectivating, acquisitive functions of conscious mentation upon the primary feeling sphere of existence. He postulated the principle of the infant's *primary identification* with the mother as the biological matrix of later developments in the direction of neurosis as well as of constructive societal coordination and spontaneous personality integration (1917). Even before this, Burrow had suggested that conflicts, defenses, and vicarious compensations are enacted not only in the individual but also within the accepted codes and conventions of normal social living (1914). He expressed this view when he wrote of the "world's neurosis" or "neurosis of the race" (1918). In other words, he drew attention to a general human problem of which the neurotic deviation of the individual is but a symptom (1926).

Briefly, then, we find in these early psychoanalytic studies themes that predominate in Burrow's later investigations, namely: (1) recognition of an inherently constructive, phylo-organismic basis of interrelatedness and personality integration; (2) complications arising from developing objectivation, consciousness, and image-symbol usage; (3) expression of the resulting conflict in social patterns of compromise and self-contradiction in which the individual is an active participant; and (4) the attempt to understand and formulate in biological terms the factors involved.

The specific event that led Burrow to extend the analytic procedure to the group setting occurred in 1918, when his student-assistant, Clarence Shields, suggested that they reverse the roles of analyst and patient. In the often arduous mutual analysis that followed, a residue of irrational self-justification and antagonism that did not yield to genetic analysis was found in each participant. The difficulty could not be fully understood in terms of historically conditioned transference and countertransference reactions, nor could it be ascribed predominantly to one or the other of the participants. Rather, they were faced with an interactive complex of self-biased attitudes, defenses, and evasions that tended to obstruct the effort to investigate the problem. It became evident that there existed an obsessively guarded impediment to contact and communication that was not limited to the specific analytic situation, but consisted rather in a general social condition that required further study (1927 a).

Under these circumstances, it was a natural step for Burrow to invite other individuals, students and patients, to participate in their joint study. Not only was this step in keeping with the evidently social nature of the problem, but there was also the possibility that the impasse could be more readily understood and resolved by extending the investigation within a larger social setting. In 1927, The Lifwynn Foundation for Laboratory Research in Analytic and Social Psychiatry was organized to sustain and sponsor these researches.

The group analytic studies that developed took place in formal laboratory meetings, in which from four to twenty "normal" and neurotic individuals participated. This social self-inquiry was also carried over into everyday professional and domestic activities the participants shared as members of the laboratory group or experimental community (Burrow, 1928 a and b; Syz, 1928; Galt, 1933).

Setting aside as far as possible conventional distinctions based on social roles and professional status, the students made a consistent attempt to bring to awareness and expression the latent content of their reactions as they occurred in the immediacy of the group interchange. They brought up for analytic evaluation, for instance, the interwoven dynamics of authoritarian and submissive attitudes, competitive self-assertion and its socially sanctioned disguises, hostility and its moralistic pretenses, seemingly altruistic though self-centered behavior, and other discrepant, predominantly unconscious trends. Such manifestations were examined not as isolated occurrences but as behavior processes embedded within the individual's self-structure, in the interaction among the various participants, and in the group as a whole. There was increasing evidence that these phenomena are dynamically related to or expressive of a common denominator, which may be characterized as *autistic image-dependence*.[6] That is, undue emphasis and dependence upon the preeminent self-image and its socially systematized projections and disguises were found to be an ever-present motive in verbal and nonverbal interchanges, active and passive manifestations, role enactments, characterological attitudes, and socially sanctioned forms of conduct. In the phenomenological analysis of emotional processes (for instance of the common anger reaction) overtly expressed or implied in the immediate group interchange, various aspects of the autistically systematized attachment to image-symbol constructs were observed as interrelated parts of a total constellation.

Thus, a variety of experiential and behavioral phenomena, whether apparently benign or disruptive, were recognized as phases of a dynamic structure that is variously actualized in intrapersonal and interpersonal processes and that has noxious implications. On the one hand, there are relations to or continuity with resentful oppositeness and detachment, with guilt and anxiety, and with the endless defensive and compensatory, symptom-producing sequels; on the other hand, we have a direct transition to outright hostile-destructive developments in their individual and social expressions. We find here a source of impeded communication and inadequate relatedness, an interference with spontaneity and the full use of inherent assets, a motive for self-assertive social cluster formations with their intergroup antagonisms. The dynamics of autistic image-bondage are expressed in the prevailing forms of education and social conditioning in which each

---

6. Eugen Bleuler introduced the term "autistic" in 1911 to characterize the wishful nature of schizophrenic thinking, which is directed by self-centered affects rather than by reality and logic. He emphasized that autistic trends also occur in other psychopathological conditions and in normal children and adults (play activities, fantasies and dreams, poetry and myths). Bleuler drew special attention to the distorting effect of autistic thinking upon medical theory and practice (1919). I use the term *autistic image-dependence* to characterize the dynamic trend in self-structure and social interaction that is intensively preoccupied with and dependent upon the defense of the self-image, experienced as a detached entity that is potentially opposed to or hostile to other humans and the outside world.

child is trained to respond to right-wrong signals used for parental convenience, as a promise of love and protection, and as a mutual defense of personal advantage and distinction. These educational techniques tend to perpetuate a dynamic structure in the individual and society through which the *appearance* of social interest is employed for unacknowledged competitive interests and self-centered defenses.

An especially noteworthy manifestation of this urge to defend the self-image is its distorting influence upon perception and observation. That is, the material to be observed may be so closely related to the process of observation that a sober evaluation of its structure is impeded. Not only are one's own socially undesirable trends kept out of the perceptual field, but the autistically oriented cognitive function tends to reinforce the limited, self-centered perspective it was supposed to observe and evaluate.

Our group-analytic observations, then, indicated that we are confronted with a socially structured behavioral defect, whose dynamics embody important etiological or causative factors. That is, we deal not only with a general neurotogenic disposition that under adverse conditions may lead to behavior disorders, but there is also a socio-individual configuration (Syz, 1930) that in itself generates antisocial and morbid action formations. This affectosymbolic systematization, designated by Burrow as the *'I'-persona* (1937), was considered by him all along as a maladaptive structure that is institutionalized in terms of interrelational values and conduct (*the social neurosis*) (1918, 1927 a). The terms *phylobiology, phylopathology,* and *phyloanalysis* (Burrow 1930, 1937; Galt, 1933; Riese, 1963; Syz, 1946, 1963) were introduced by him as available data indicated that the psychophysiological processes involved are characteristic of human nature generally and not specific to particular personality organizations or cultural patterns. In Burrow's studies, the analysis of these socially structured neurotogenic trends always proceeded from the background of a vital recognition of man's integrative, phylo-organismic capacity.

The above-mentioned obstruction to adequate observation and analysis was intensively worked with throughout the group-analytic investigations, and the observer was consistently included as an interactive part of the condition studied. Burrow discussed this feature in *The Social Basis of Consciousness* (1927 a) and in many papers published prior to 1930, and emphasized the necessity of establishing through common social analysis a *consensual basis of observation* (1925). This term indicated that, from the basis of the mutual challenge of the personal affect-bias, it should become possible to appraise in an increasingly objective manner the socially constellated behavior defect in which each observer participated.

Since Burrow's early work, much has been written about participant observation and consensual validation in psychiatric as well as in sociological contexts. We find concern with the observer's or therapist's position in the discussions regarding countertransference, and in psychology we have the transactional movement, in which the knower and the known are included in a common system (Cantril et al., 1949; Dewey and Bentley, 1949). Studies on cultural relativity show a similar emphasis, and there is a parallel movement in modern physics in which the observer and the observed are no longer considered as independent entities (Heisenberg, 1958).

However, what Burrow and his coworkers tried to do was more specific. They made an effort to include consistently the observer's socially sanctioned autistic trend. Unless this trend is specifically taken into account, so-called consensual validation may lead to a compounding of personal bias rather than to its elimination. On the other hand, if our findings are correct, inclusion of the socially structured impediment in which we, as therapists and investigators, also participate may be a significant step toward developing an adequate perspective for value judgments in the field of mental and social health.[7] In our investigations, Burrow's consensual observation came to be combined with the specific proprioceptive measures discussed in the next section of this essay.

It is perhaps not surprising that Burrow's group work was often misunderstood or vigorously opposed when he presented it at psychiatric and psychoanalytic meetings in the twenties and thirties. It is an interesting social phenomenon that later on, when certain aspects of his trend were incorporated in psychiatric and group psychotherapeutic practice, his pioneer efforts remained almost completely unacknowledged. There was considerable, and often justified, criticism of the difficulty of his writings and of certain concepts he proposed. I suggest, however, that there was also—and still is—an emotionally defensive feature in the response to his unorthodox and uncompromising extension of the analysis to the structure and the defenses of the socially adapted self. I know from my own experience how powerful these resistances are and how resourceful one's own self is in finding justification for warding off what appears to be an intrusion upon one's established security and rightness. We should also admit that the human dilemma that Burrow tried to bring to awareness and investiga-

---

7. In my therapeutic work with neurotic patients ("inclusive psychotherapy") I found it very helpful to emphasize, conceptually and operationally, the socio-individual structure of self-reference and its associated dynamics, in which the therapist himself is also involved (1936, 1957).

tion, namely, man's self-destructive trend lodged in his habitual self-identify, is indeed a difficult problem—difficult to realize, to formulate, and to work with on the scientific level. Concern with this problem may interrupt in a disturbing manner the routine of our days, the theoretical refinement of established though perhaps erroneous concepts, and our preoccupation with the intricacies of therapeutic pursuits. However, it appears that the demands of our rapidly changing culture, with its revisions of accepted common sense, may so modify our frame of reference that the broader issue of man's self-defeating involvements will become a legitimate and urgent object of scientific inquiry.

Insofar as group psychotherapies consist of an insightful reorientation occurring in group interaction, it seems that Burrow's group analysis was the only forerunner of such psychotherapies in this country. However, there are distinctive features that characterize Burrow's group analysis and differentiate it from the group psychotherapies that developed later, namely, (1) emphasis upon research, (2) the altered frame of reference that centers upon the neurotogenic aspects of the normal reaction average from the background of phylo-organismic conceptions, (3) consistent inclusion of the observer's own autistic trend, and (4) the employment of proprioceptive measures for bringing about a reorientation of attitude and insight. Though therapeutic changes occurred among the participants in group analysis (such as improved communication, lessened dependence on parent images, and a release of constructive forces), the dominant interest was in developing concepts and measures that would mobilize healthy function by eliminating destructive or immature involvements, not only in neurotic individuals but also in the community generally.

PROPRIOCEPTIVE ASPECTS

In the late 1920s Burrow (1930) and his associates began developing proprioceptive experimentation. The group-analytic investigations had resulted in a fuller awareness and understanding of the essential inter-relational problem but had not led to a resolution of it. The unremitting observation of self-referent attitudes and affects, with its challenge of accustomed values and incentives, constituted a painfully frustrating experience. At the same time, the terms of the group experiment precluded recourse to the usual evasive devices. In this condition of affect challenge and frustration, Burrow unexpectedly became aware of tensional sensations in the oculofacial region that appeared to be significantly related to the affectosymbolic blockage.

That is, the shift of attention to the perception of strains in the fore-part of the head was accompanied by a change of attitude or emotional orientation that tended to resolve the affective impasse. At first, these sensations were only fleeting and elusive, and readily gave way to customary affect preoccupations. However, with consistent practice, in which several of Burrow's associates participated, the sense of stress in the ocular and frontal areas came more readily to awareness. In the procedure developed and recommended by Burrow, the eyes were kept, as far as possible, in a relaxed and steady position. This balance in ocular function was to be maintained solely through internal kinesthetic sensation. In the course of this proprioceptive experimentation, the localized tensional patterns were sensed increasingly against the tensional pattern perceptible throughout the organism as a whole. Or one might say that a mergence occurred between the local and the total tensional patterns, in which the total pattern assumed dominance.

As mentioned above, the shift of attentional focus or awareness from behavioral imagery to the "feeling-sensation" of endoorganismic patterns went along with a shift in the total behavioral constellation. This behavioral change consisted in an elimination or reduction of habitual image preoccupations and self-referent affects such as elation, irritation, guilt, regret, and other forms of self-justification. This shift was accompanied by an inclusive feeling-contact with others and a sense of internal ease. Perhaps one could say that the lessened impetus to protect favorable self-appraisals went along with liberation of an organismically rooted integration and interrelational connectedness. Thus, the adaptive defect, which had been previously worked with on the behavioral level, could now be approached by a proprioceptive technique. That is, an altered value orientation was established that was not primarily based on conceptual interpretation.

On the basis of these observations Burrow began to distinguish between two attentional modes: *ditention,* or the customary self-reflective and defensive mode of adaptation, and *cotention,* in which the orientation to one's kind and to the world is direct and organismically integrated (1941). There were indications that with continued practice the cotentive mode could be carried into everyday activities, thus affecting behavior and interrelational contact in the direction of increasing societal coordination.

With regard to the interpretation of the psychophysiological factors involved in the proprioceptive experimentation, one might postulate that the tensional sensations relate to incipient motor innervations and that the attitudinal changes observed rest on a reorganization of such motor configurations. The motor patterns in the oculofacial region are especially engaged in our contact with the environment through verbal and nonverbal functions, and they appear especially involved in the affectosymbolic systematization of the self as it interacts with its social world. Where there is kinesthetic awareness of the mergence of localized motor innervations with the organism's total motor pattern—where the local oculofacial pattern is sensed from the background of total proprioceptive awareness—we may assume that this reconstellation in the hierarchy of motor innervations would be reflected in a shift of feeling, mental attitude, and action.

This interpretation of an interrelation between kinesthetic components and behavior falls in with the "motor theories of consciousness" that have been advocated since the end of the last century by a number of investigators. The important role of incipient motor patterns in the structure of psychological phenomena has been indicated in experiments by Nina Bull (1951), who concluded that preparatory motor patterns and associated visceral innervations are basic ingredients in emotion, goal orientation, and mental content.[8]

Against this background we can more readily understand the interrelations between (1) the integration of the endoorganismic sensations referred to, (2) the reconstellation of preparatory motor innervations reinforced by proprioceptive feedback, and (3) the corresponding change in feeling, attitude, evaluation and action. These are all interrelated aspects of a total process throughout the personality structure. On this basis one can suggest a comprehensive conceptual system that includes physiological, psychological, and social phases of behavior, as well as introspective and proprioceptive aspects of experience. In our experimentation, the reconstellation meant a total shift from autistically deflected attention (ditention) to an inclusive, societally oriented attitude and feeling (cotention).

Burrow and his associates tried to determine specifically some of the physiological factors associated with these changes of orientation. Through instrumental recordings, we found in cotention (1) a markedly slowed and deepened respiratory rhythm, (2) a decrease in frequency and range of eye movements, and (3) a decrease in the alpha component as well as in the amplitude of electrical brain waves (Burrow, 1950, pp. 353–392). With respect to respiration, it was of interest to find that, while the minute-volume of air inspired in cotention was significantly less than in ditention, the average amount of oxygen

---

8. For a fuller consideration of the possible role of incipient motor activations in attitude, self-identity, and emotion, see also Bally, 1933, and Syz, 1963, pp. 76–78.

actually absorbed in the cotentive and ditentive conditions was about the same; that is, the percentage of oxygen utilized in the inspired air was considerably higher in cotention than in ditention. We did not find consistent differences in pulse rate, blood pressure, and cardiac activity.

I have no interpretation to offer that would relate these physiological modifications specifically to the attentional changes, other than to point out that the function of breathing is, of course, essential for maintaining the organism's homeostasis and growth. It mediates on a basic biological level man's interrelation, or rather his continuity, with the environment. On the behavioral level, breathing expresses specific attitudes to the world, and is an essential element in communication through speech. With regard to eye movements, they not only play an important role in thinking and imagination, but also serve as an essential tool in guiding the organism's orientation. Both the visual and the respiratory apparatus—like behavior generally—are controlled by autonomic as well as cerebrospinal innervations. Thus, these functions can be regarded as sensitive reagents to differing behavioral events, and it is understandable that they reflect also the differences in the total adaptive constellation characterized here by the terms ditention and cotention.

DISCUSSION

With regard to the interpretation of the socially systematized behavior defect that we investigated from the background of our own participation in it, Burrow's emphasis all along was on a group, or phylocentric, point of view. That is, the individual was considered as an integrated part, in feeling and action, of the community as a whole. In an extension of his early psychoanalytic formulations, Burrow postulated an evolutional miscarriage coincident with the development of man's elaborate symbol and language usage. He suggested that organismic drives and total feeling processes had been mischanneled into the cortical and cephalic regions, and that there had thus occurred an upsurge of basic organismic impulses into the symbolic segment. In this way a divisive self-identity developed; that is, an internal decentration or conflict occurred in which total feeling and organismic forces became unduly attached to symbolic part-features of the social environment and of the self. An unjustified sense of self-eminence developed, and a world of self-centered individuals was created in which each insists on his esoteric rightness. But while Burrow emphasized socioindividual totality and the emergence of conflict within man as a species in the course of evolution, he also placed great stress on noxious social conditioning.

It may be added that dynamic aspects of the symbol-affect systematization or "misappropriation" of feeling have a relation to the early omnipotent phase, in which signals and words assume for the child a magic power in managing his world and in which, through identification with these signals, the self-identity is endowed with inordinate power. Another dynamic feature may be traced to the transformation of the child's early biological dependence into dependence upon the parent image, which begins to play an important role in internal as well as in interindividual adjustments. This dependence upon individually and socially systematized images, reinforced by conditioning, is injurious in its autistic structure as well as in the exaggerated anchoring on peripheral image-symbol constructs. For a fuller understanding of this socioindividual impasse it will be necessary to consider it in relation to a model of essential human characteristics. While I shall not enter into these aspects of our problem, I should like to emphasize that accumulating scientific evidence permits us to go beyond a merely intuitive and personally biased image of man's nature (Syz, 1957, sections IV and V).

In the psychotherapeutic setting, the socially patterned malfunction finds its expression in the interlaced complex of transference and countertransference reactions. On the basis of our phyloanalytic observations, transference is a pervasive, immature, and neurotogenic reaction pattern that is ever present in everyday interchanges as well as in therapeutic transactions (Burrow 1927 b). While not disregarding the more acute involvements of transference interaction, we are especially interested in investigating the essential nature of the self-referent type of interrelationship. In addition to the restrictive influence upon the therapeutic process, autistic image-dependence (or what might be called pervasive transference) leads to an overemphasis on individual details of neurotic involvements and to an inadequate recognition of socially sanctioned defenses, that is, of the larger social ineptitude that is dynamically interlinked with the individual disorder.

I would like to add a few comments regarding other investigations that may be compared with Burrow's approach to the human problem. While the somewhat vague idea of "social pathology" has been applied to a variety of noxious social situations, researches in social psychiatry and cultural anthropology, as previously mentioned, attempt to determine more specifically the sociocultural value and action patterns that have a damaging effect on behavioral health.

There are a number of trends or theories that in one way or another show similarities to Burrow's position. His early emphasis on

divisiveness and detachment due to the inappropriate use of objectivating and symbolic functions has parallels in the existentialist concern
about the alienation of man from society and from himself. This
alienation is ascribed to exaggerated symbolic mentation and concomitant exclusion of feeling participation. In Buber's philosophy,
man's present condition is considered as a form of disease (1948).
In his interpretation, mind has become separated from instinct and
body. Man has not yet found the new position that is specific to him
as a human being and that permits a real meeting with others.

The German psychologist and philosopher Ludwig Klages con-
trasted a *biocentric* position with the *logocentric* attitude that, in his
view, has developed in the last two thousand years, and that he considered the major cause of the present impoverishment and deterioration of human nature. Klages (1929–1932) wrote extensively about
these problems, but did not suggest any remedial steps.

The movement of General Semantics, introduced by A. Korzybski
(1933), also deals with a general disorder in human adjustment or
evaluation that is ascribed to a false use of symbols, namely, to an
erroneous identification of words or linguistic symbols with the materials or processes for which they stand. Korzybski pointed out the
extent to which the verbal concept is projected into the perception of
the thing itself. A confusion of different orders of abstraction thus
occurs, resulting in various behavioral troubles and aggravated by the
fact that many linguistic forms are static and elementalistic rather
than flexible and dynamic. The aim of General Semantics is to bring
about consciousness of abstracting, which is considered to be an important first step towards a far-going reorientation in which the structure of linguistic usage is in accordance with the structure of the universe and of the nervous system. However, this procedure does not
include in its challenge the socially systematized self-identity that
was the focus of Burrow's studies.

In an early review, L. L. Whyte (1929) referred to Burrow's
"revolutionary view that not only the 'neurotic' but the 'normal' civilized man is in the grip of a mental dissociation." He later elaborated
this theme in his own way (1948), and gave a historical-descriptive
account of what he considered the dualistic tradition that developed
in man's evolution and that interferes with biological coordination.
Whyte expressed the view that at present we are in a phase of growing awareness and realization of the formative processes that unite
man with nature; that is, there are indications of a unitary reorganization.

Erich Fromm (1955) proposed the concept of a "socially patterned
defect" expressed in normal individuals who, living in abstractions,

have become alienated from things, people, and themselves. The individual who cannot accept this socially prevalent pattern is apt to develop a clinical neurotic disorder. This defect, according to Fromm, has developed in the Western world in the last few centuries due to increasing industrialization, mechanization, and marketing orientation. As a remedy, he suggested the development of external sociocultural adjustments, a "communitarian socialism" that, together with a reorientation in attitude and character structure, should lead to the attainment of sanity and mental health.

Neither Whyte nor Fromm specifically takes account of the observer's (that is, our own) involvement in the social defect to which they refer. This is one aspect in which they differ from Burrow. Also, the dissociation they describe would seem to take up only partial aspects of the general human problem with which Burrow was concerned.

From the point of view of biology; Bertalanffy (1958) proposed that while the symbol world makes of man a human being, it is at the same time the cause of the bloody course of history. Only within the framework of ideologies can we understand warfare. The neurotic dilemma seems to arise from conflicts between a symbol universe and biological drives, or between opposing symbol worlds. However, the symbolic structures of social convention, morals, religions, and various forms of sublimation may be able to check the aggressive tendency in man.

In his later years, Freud himself began to be interested in the sociological aspects of behavior disorders. In *Civilization and Its Discontents* (1930) he wrote, "If the evolution of civilization has such a far-reaching similarity with the development of an individual, and if the same methods are employed in both, would not the diagnosis be justified that many systems of civilization—or epochs of it—possibly even the whole of humanity—have become 'neurotic' under the pressure of the civilizing trends?" He realized that we are faced with a new and difficult situation in which the "normal" social setting is the problem, but he suggested that "In spite of all these difficulties, we may expect that one day someone will venture upon this research into the pathology of civilized communities," and that "To analytic dissection of these neuroses therapeutic recommendations might follow which could claim a great practical interest."

In his early psychoanalytic papers, Burrow had called attention to the need to extend the analytic inquiry to society as a whole (1914, 1918). In 1924, after he had started his research project in concrete group settings, he wrote, "the time is not far distant when the psychopathologist must awaken to his wider function of clinical sociologist and recognize his obligation to challenge the neurosis in its social as well as in its individual intrenchments" (p. 235). Freud, although acquainted with these group analytic undertakings (letter of January 28, 1925, in Burrow, 1958, p. 85), did not concur with Burrow's method of applying analytic methods to the social problem (Burrow, 1950, p. xiv), and later, when he "came upon the category of the mankind neurosis" (Binswanger, 1956, p. 115), he did not refer to Burrow's earlier emphasis upon the same theme.

With regard to therapeutic recommendations, Herbert Read wrote (1949), "Only Trigant Burrow has suggested a *method,* even a technique, by means of which our social aberrations can be corrected. . . . Essentially what Dr. Burrow is proposing is not a psychological experiment, but new foundations for the next phase in human evolution."

Other analytically oriented investigators have expressed ideas related to Burrow's concepts, for instance, Jung's concept of the collective unconscious, Adler's emphasis on striving for superiority and the concomitant neglect of social feeling, and Horney's ideas concerning neurotic pride and self-idealization. Kubie (1957) postulated that a "neurotic potential" is universal because of the special role symbolic functions play in human development. Out of this neurotic potential a "neurotic process" evolves that in some degree is ever present. "Distortion of the symbolic function" and the predominance of unconscious processes are important factors that, under appropriate circumstances, may lead to the "neurotic state" (outspoken behavior pathology). Important sociocultural influences on these processes, according to Kubie, are inadequately understood.[9]

Further, from the background of Burrow's studies one would question the adequacy of evaluations and conceptions that accept as basic a personality or self-system that rests largely on reflected self-appraisals and security operations (Sullivan, 1945), or on the drive to enhance and secure the symbolic or phenomenological self (Snygg and Combs, 1949). We would ask, rather, to what extent the actual

---

9. More recently, R. D. Laing (1967) has taken the position that "what we call 'normal' is a product of repression, denial, splitting, projection, introjection and other forms of destructive action to experience." These socially shared processes are expressed in the prevailing, normal form of alienation that has to be taken into account in our approach to forms of alienation that are less frequent and relatively strange and are "labeled by the 'normal' majority as bad or mad." As we are all implicated in the state of alienation, "psychotherapy must remain *an obstinate attempt of two people to recover the wholeness of being human through the relationship between them.*"

predominance of these defensive systems in personality and culture, and the emphasis placed upon them in theoretical formulations, are an expression of a general bias toward a neurotic type of adaptation.

In the comparative consideration of the above-mentioned views and methods, one has to take into account that Burrow envisioned the problem from a comprehensively phyletic background. Group analytic experience led him also to include investigations of the autistic image accentuation in "normal" interaction and embodied in himself. As he emphasized, mere intellectual or verbal acknowledgment of self-involvement cannot substitute for the observer's felt awareness of his participation in the reaction tissue observed. This self-inclusion may make it possible to submit pervasive socioindividual malfunction to scientific investigation. The beginning made in this direction in phylo-biological investigation included the beginning of a reintegrative process that may counter noxious trends.

Turning to possible comparisons with the proprioceptive technique, a few other methods use somatizing measures, and in a way may confirm certain aspects of Burrow's work with tensional patterns. Hefferline (1958), Jacobson (1929), and others have recorded muscular tension electromyographically and have related kinesthetic awareness to certain behavior phenomena. Of special interest are the observations by Malmo and Smith (1954–1955), who ask whether tension in the frontalis muscle can be taken as an index of "emotionality." Perls, Hefferline, and Goodman (1951) have included proprioceptive aspects of experience in the therapeutic system termed Gestalt Therapy. But their inclusion of proprioceptive patterns is not specifically oriented toward the socially structured deflection of attention upon the autistic self-image.

Edmund Jacobson (1929) showed in his experimental studies, in some of which he recorded muscular tensions by action currents, the close relation of muscular activation to imagery, thinking, and emotion. He developed a technique of "progressive relaxation," which proved of therapeutic value in many neurotic conditions. In our studies of internal tensional patterns, the shift from ditention to cotention was not accomplished by inducing general motor relaxation, although a factor of decreased muscular tonus may be involved in the proprioceptive reintegration that took place.

Another widely used somatizing approach is the "concentrative self-relaxation" on which J. H. Schultz has reported since 1932 in detailed publications under the title *Das Autogene Training* (1956). A guided self-training program proceeds through six standard exercises and leads to a submergence into bodily sensations that makes it possible to influence consciously various functions such as muscle tonus, heartbeat, and blood circulation, as well as certain emotional trends.[10]

Burrow's experimentation differs from this method in that it deals specifically with the sensing of oculofacial patterns of tension and their relation to the organism's total tensional configuration. It does not include the fargoing submergence in bodily sensations, nor the autosuggestive control of disturbing habits as emphasized by Schultz in his technique of autorelaxation. The interest focuses not on the elimination of certain symptoms of tension, anxiety, or emotional overreaction in the individual neurotic, but rather on the development of an altered attitudinal orientation that takes into account, and may prove effective in dealing with, man's basic interrelational disorder.

There is another large area that does not employ customary psychotherapeutic measures but in which bodily involvement is an important factor. I refer to the various teachings and techniques that have been practiced in the East, especially to the Zen procedures, which have a long tradition and which in recent years have aroused much interest in Western countries. While I have had no direct contact with the Zen method, it appears that its aim is to overcome the customary self-oriented mode and to reach a more direct type of experience and action. Some exponents of this method see a similarity with Burrow's shift to cotention and other aspects of his thesis (Tomita, 1956; Watts, 1958).[11]

It is clear from the foregoing comments that there are similarities and parallels to the phylobiological position in a number of methods, schools, and theories. Nevertheless, Burrow's integrating of self-inclusive inquiry, endoorganismic perception, and species orientation, in the setting of a research endeavor, appears to be distinctive and offers a comprehensive perspective for the reappraisal of human values. From this basis, significant criteria of mental health may be formulated in terms of a dynamically integrative constellation that favors constructive relatedness and creative growth in individual and group.

---

10. *Autogenic Therapy*, a six-volume series, was edited by Luthe (1969–1973) partly in cooperation with Schultz. It treats medical and psychotherapeutic applications, research and theory, and the dynamics of "autogenic neutralization."

11. In the last ten or fifteen years there has been an upsurge of interest in a variety of techniques that reduce customary mentation and mobilize the organism's nonverbal resources. For a discussion of the range of these procedures, see, for instance, Hanna (1973). Benson, Beary, and Carol (1974) proposed that self-induced shifts may be based on an integrated central nervous system reaction ("relaxation response"). The relation of Burrow's phyloanalytic method to some of these techniques, particularly "sensory awareness," has been considered by A. S. Galt (1973), who also called attention to similarities and differences between Burrow's group-analysis and current group approaches.

References

Allport, G. W., "The Trend in Motivational Theory," *American Journal of Orthopsychiatry, 23:* 107–119, 1953.

Angyal, A., *Foundation for a Science of Personality* (New York: The Commonwealth Fund, 1941; Viking, 1972).

Arensberg, C., "Values in Action," *Human Organization, 17:25–26,* 1958.

Bally, G., "Die frühkindliche Motorik im Vergleich mit der Motorik der Tiere," *Imago, 19:339–366,* 1933.

Benson, H., Beary, J. F., and Carol, M. P., "The Relaxation Response," *Psychiatry, 37:37–46,* 1974.

Bertalanffy, L. von, "The Theory of Open Systems in Physics and Biology," *Science, 111:23–29,* 1950.

———, "Comments on Aggression," *Bulletin of the Menninger Clinic, 22:* 50–57, 1958.

Bertalanffy, L. von, and Woodger, J. H., *Modern Theories of Development, An Introduction to Theoretical Biology* (London: Oxford University Press, 1933).

Bidney, D., "Human Nature and the Cultural Process," *American Anthropologist, 49:375–396,* 1947.

Binswanger, L., *Erinnerungen an Sigmund Freud* (Bern: Francke, 1956).

Bleuler, E., *Dementia Praecox, or The Group of Schizophrenias* (New York: International Universities Press, 1950; appeared in 1911 as a volume of Aschaffenburg's *Handbuch*).

———, *Das Autistisch-Undisziplinierte Denken in der Medizin und Seine Überwindung* (Berlin: Julius Springer, 1919).

Bridgman, P. W., "Philosophical Implications of Physics," *American Academy of Sciences Bulletin,* 1950, vol. 3, no. 5.

Buber, M., *Das Problem des Menschen* (Heidelberg: Schneider, 1948).

Bull, N., *The Attitude Theory of Emotion* (New York: Coolidge Foundation, Nervous and Mental Disease Monographs, 1951).

Burrow, T. "The Psychanalyst and the Community," *Journal of the American Medical Association, 62:1876–1878,* 1914.

———, "The Genesis and Meaning of 'Homosexuality' and Its Relation to the Problem of Introverted Mental States," *Psychoanalytic Review, 4:272–284,* 1917.

———, "The Origin of the Incest-Awe," *Psychoanalytic Review, 5:243–254,* 1918.

———, "Social Images Versus Reality," *Journal of Abnormal Psychology and Social Psychology, 19:230–235,* 1924.

———, "Psychiatry as an Objective Science," *British Journal of Medical Psychology, 5:298–309,* 1925.

———, "Insanity a Social Problem," *American Journal of Sociology, 32:* 80–87, 1926.

———, (a) *The Social Basis of Consciousness* (New York: Harcourt 1927).

———, (b) "The Problem of the Transference," *British Journal of Medical Psychology, 7:193–202,* 1927.

————, (a) "The Basis of Group-Analysis, or the Analysis of the Reactions of Normal and Neurotic Individuals," *British Journal of Medical Psychology*, 8:198–206, 1928.

————, (b) "The Autonomy of the 'I' from the Standpoint of Group Analysis," *Psyche*, 8:35–50, 1928.

————, "Physiological Behavior-Reactions in the Individual and the Community: A Study in Phyloanalysis," *Psyche*, 11:67–81, 1930.

————, *The Biology of Human Conflict*, (New York: Macmillan, 1937).

————, "Kymograph Records of Neuromuscular (Respiratory) Patterns in Relation to Behavior Disorders," *Psychosomatic Medicine*, 3:174–186, 1941.

————, *The Neurosis of Man* (New York: Harcourt-Brace, 1950; reprinted in: *Science and Man's Behavior*, New York: Philosophical Library, 1953).

————, *A Search for Man's Sanity—The Selected Letters of Trigant Burrow, with Biographical Notes* (New York: Oxford University Press, 1958).

Cantril, H.; Ames, A., Jr.; Hastorf, A. H.; and Ittelson, W. H., "Psychology and Scientific Research," *Science*, 110:461–464, 491–497, 517–522, 1949.

Cofer, C. N. and Appley, M. H., *Motivation: Theory and Research* (New York: John Wiley and Sons, 1965).

Conant, J. B., *Modern Science and Modern Man* (Garden City, N.Y.: Doubleday-Anchor, 1953).

Darwin, C., *Expressions of the Emotions in Man and Animals* (New York: Appleton, 1916; first published in 1872).

Dewey, J. and Bentley, A. F., *Knowing and the Known* (Boston: Beacon Press, 1949).

Edel, A., "Concept of Values in Contemporary Philosophical Values Theory," *Philosophy of Science*, 20:198–207, 1953.

Emerson, A. E., "Dynamic Homeostasis: A Unifying Principle in Organic, Social, and Ethical Evolution," *Scientific Monthly*, 78:67–85, 1954.

Freud, S., *Civilization and Its Discontents* (London: Hogarth Press, 1951; first published 1930).

Fromm, E. *The Sane Society* (New York: Rinehart, 1955).

Galt, A. S., "Therapy in the Context of Trigant Burrow's Group Analysis," *Group Process*, 5:115–128, 1973.

Galt, W., "Phyloanalysis—A Brief Study, in Trigant Burrow's Group or Phyletic Method of Behavior Analysis," *Journal of Abnormal and Social Psychology*, 27:411–429, 1933.

Gerard, R. W., "A Biological Basis for Ethics: The Attack on Science," *Philosophy of Science*, 9:92–120, 1942.

———— ed., "Concepts of Biology," *Behavioral Science*, 3:103–196, 1958.

Goldenweiser, A., "The Autonomy of the Social," *American Anthropologist*, 19:447–449, 1917.

Goldstein, K., *The Organism—A Holistic Approach to Biology* (New York: American Book Company, 1939).

————, "Organismic Approach to the Problem of Motivation," *Transactions of the New York Academy of Science*, 9:218–230, 1947.

Grinker, R. R., ed., *Toward a Unified Theory of Human Behavior* (New York: Basic Books, 1956).

Hanna, T., "The Project of Somatology," *Journal of Humanistic Psychology*, 13:3–14, 1973.

Hefferline, R. F., "The Role of Proprioception in the Control of Behavior," *Transactions of the New York Academy of Sciences*, 20:739–764, 1958.

Heisenberg, W., *Physics and Philosophy* (New York: Harper and Brothers, 1958).

Herrick, C. J., "Biological Determinism and Human Freedom," *International Journal of Ethics*, 37:36–52, 1926.

Jacobson, E., *Progressive Relaxation* (Chicago: University of Chicago Press, 1929).

Jahoda, M., *Current Concepts of Positive Mental Health* (New York: Basic Books, 1958).

Klages, L., *Der Geist als Widersacher der Seele* (Leipzig: J. A. Barth, 1929–1932, 3 volumes).

Kluckhohn, C., "Values and Value-Orientations in the Theory of Action," in *Toward a General Theory of Action*, T. Parsons and E. A. Shils, eds. (Cambridge: Harvard University Press, 1954).

Korzybski, A., *Science and Sanity* (New York: International Non-Aristotelian Library, 1933).

Kroeber, A. L., "The Superorganic," *American Anthropologist*, 19:163–213, 1917.

Kubie, L. S., "Social Forces and the Neurotic Process," in *Explorations in Social Psychiatry* (New York: Basic Books, 1957).

Kuhn, T. S., *The Structure of Scientific Revolutions* (Chicago: University of Chicago Press, 1962; second enlarged edition, 1970).

Laing, R. D., *The Politics of Experience* (New York: Pantheon, 1967).

Leighton, A. H., *The Stirling County Study of Psychiatric Disorder and Sociocultural Environment* (New York: Basic Books, three volumes, 1959–1963).

Lepley, R., ed., *Value: A Cooperative Inquiry* (New York: Columbia University Press, 1949).

Luthe, W., ed., *Autogenic Therapy* (New York: Grune and Stratton, 1969–1973, six volumes).

Malmo, R. B. and Smith, A. R., "Forehead Tension and Motor Irregularities in Psychoneurotic Patients under Stress," *Journal of Personality*, 23:391–406, 1954–1955.

Maslow, A. H., ed., *New Knowledge in Human Values* (New York: Harper Brothers, 1959).

Morris, C., *Varieties of Human Value* (Chicago: University of Chicago Press, 1956).

Murray, H. A. and Morgan, C. D., "A Clinical Study of Sentiments," *Genetic Psychology Monographs*, 32:5–149, 155–311, 1945.

Offer, D. and Sabshin, M., *Normality: Theoretical and Clinical Concepts of Mental Health* (New York: Basic Books, 1966).

Opler, M. K., *Culture, Psychiatry, and Human Values* (Springfield, Ill.: Charles C. Thomas, 1956).

Perls, F. S.; Hefferline, R. F.; and Goodman, P., *Gestalt Therapy* (New York: Julian Press, 1951).

Perry, R. B., *Realms of Value* (Cambridge: Harvard University Press, 1954).

Read, H., "Burrow's *The Neurosis of Man*" (review), *The Tiger's Eye, 1*: 115–117, 1949.

Redlich, F. C., "The Concept of Normality," *American Journal of Psychotherapy, 6*:551–576, 1952.

Riese, W., *L'Ideé de l'Homme dans la Neurologie Contemporaine*, (Paris: Alcan, 1938).

———, "The Principle of Integration," *Journal of Nervous and Mental Disease, 96*:296–312, 1942.

———, *The Conception of Disease: Its History, Its Versions, and Its Nature* (New York: Philosophical Library, 1953).

———, "Phyloanalysis (Burrow)—Its Historical and Philosophical Implications," in *Phyloanalysis: Theoretical and Practical Considerations on Burrow's Group-Analytic and Socio-Therapeutic Method, Supplement to Acta Psychotherapeutica, 11*:5–36, 1963.

Sapir, E., "Do We Need a 'Superorganic'?" *American Anthropologist, 19*: 441–447, 1917.

Schrödinger, E., *Science and Humanism: Physics in Our Time* (Cambridge: University Press, 1952).

Schultz, J. H., *Das Autogene Training (Konzentrative Selbstentspannung)*, 9th edition (Stuttgart: Georg Thieme Verlag), 1956).

Sinnott, E. W., *The Biology of the Spirit* (New York: Viking Press, 1955).

Smith, M. B., "Optima of Mental Health," *Psychiatry, 13*:503–510, 1950.

Syngg, D. and Combs, A. W., *Individual Behavior* (New York: Harper and Brothers, 1949).

Spiro, M. E., "Human Nature in Its Psychological Dimensions," *American Anthropologist, 56*:19–30, 1954.

Srole, L.; Langner, T. S.; Michael, S. T.; Opler, M. K.; and Rennie, T. A. C., *Mental Health in the Metropolis: the Midtown Manhattan Study* (New York: McGraw Hill, 1962).

Sullivan, H. S., *Conceptions of Modern Psychiatry* (Washington, D.C.: William Alanson White Psychiatric Foundation, 1945).

Syz, H., "Remarks on Group Analysis," *American Journal of Psychiatry, 8*:141–148, 1928.

———, "Socio-Individual Principles in Psychopathology," *British Journal of Medical Psychology, 10*:329–343, 1930.

———, "The Concept of the Organism-as-a-Whole and Its Application to Clinical Situations," *Human Biology, 8*:489–507, 1936.

———, "Phylopathology," in *Encyclopedia of Psychology*, P. L. Harriman, ed. (New York: Philosophical Library, 1946).

————, "An Experiment in Inclusive Psychotherapy," in *Experimental Psychopathology*, P. H. Hoch and J. Zubin, eds. (New York: Grune and Stratton, 1957).

————, "Reflections on Group- or Phylo-Analysis," in *Phyloanalysis: Theoretical and Practical Considerations on Burrow's Group-Analytic and Socio-Therapeutic Method, Supplement to Acta Psychotherapeutica, 11:37–88*, 1963.

————, *Vom Sein und vom Sinn* (Zurich: Editio Academica, TVZ, 1972).

Thibaut, J. W., "The Concept of Normality in Clinical Psychology," *Psychological Review, 50*:338–344, 1943.

Tomita, G., "Satori, or Buddhistic Attainment of Salvation, and the Burrowian Concept 'Cotention,'" *Tokyo Journal of Psychoanalysis, 14*:1–2, 1956.

von Monakow, C., "Die Syneidesis, das Biologische Gewissen," *Schweizer Archiv für Neurologie und Psychiatrie, 20*:56–91, 1927.

Watts, A., *Nature, Man, and Woman* (New York: Pantheon Books, 1958).

Weiss, P., in "Concepts of Biology," by R. W. Gerard, ed., *Behavioral Science, 3*:103–196, 1958.

Whitehorn, J. C., "The Scope of Motivation in Psychopathology and Psychotherapy," *American Journal of Psychoanalysis, 14*:30–39, 1954.

Whyte, L. L., "Trigant Burrow's *The Social Basis of Consciousness*" (review), *New Adelphi*, 273–275, 1929.

————, *The Next Development in Man* (New York: Henry Holt, 1948).

F. *Lhermitte and J. L. Signoret*

16

Representations and Aphasia

When Broca postulated in 1861 that a cerebral lesion localized in the third frontal convolution causes loss of speech, or aphemia, he was considering only the phonatory realization of speech. When Wernicke in 1874 showed the role of the left temporal region in verbal comprehension, he brought in the notion of auditory verbal images. And yet, Trousseau, who created the term aphasia, had emphasized the presence of a more global intellectual disturbance. Finkelnburg resolved the ensuing debate in 1870 by introducing the idea of asymbolia: Verbal disorder is, in fact, only one aspect of a more global disturbance involving all the cerebral processes that imply the use of signs, verbal or otherwise. These first years in the history of aphasia presaged the interpretations that were to be proposed in an attempt to determine the relation between thought and speech.

The concept of representation appears as a possible intermediary between cognitive functions on the one hand and verbal messages on the other. Should this representation, the perceptible content of thought, then be considered as a simple mental image, the reproduction of an anterior perception, or rather as a symbol that replaces something else?

This may seem an arbitrary distinction, since every image is already a symbol, and every symbol can possibly evoke a mental image. In any case, it is noteworthy that the evolution of ideas on aphasia has followed that concerning the relation between image and thought: "The image is the whole thought; the image is outside of all thought; the image is a moment, a fragment, an aspect of thought" (Meyerson, 1932).

When, in 1870, Fritsch and Hitzig presented experimental proof of cerebral localizations by showing that electrical excitation of the anterior part of the hemispheric convexity of a dog provokes motor activity, the theory of mental life still depended on sensualism and associationism, according to which thought is a montage binding together sensations and images or traces of sensation. It was then hypothesized that there exist depositary "centers" of these traces, the excitation of which produces images. Combined with preceding ideas, the anatomical notion (Meynert, 1867) of fibers of "association" connecting different hemispheric regions formed the basis of the associationist and geometric period of aphasia. Four centers of association were described: acoustic verbal, visual verbal, phonic or glossokinesthetic, and graphic or chirokinesthetic. Impairment of one or more of the centers, or of their associative pathways, made possible an understanding of observed disorders.

From these conceptions, two fundamental facts should be retained: (1) Aphasia should not be considered a univocal disorder, even if the acoustic verbal center does seem the most important. (2) The aphasic disorder does not depend upon a disturbance of thought. Yet, while the functional importance of the four individualized regions remains incontestable, it should be noted that the associative notion covered two fields, one referring to a theory of thought that involved an abusive conception of images, the other referring to an anatomical description that remains quite sound since it is based on connections between different cerebral regions. The isolated interruption of these connections by pathological processes enabled Wernicke to hypothesize one type of aphasia, conductive aphasia, which has since been confirmed (in particular by Geschwind, 1965). The abandonment of images resulted in a sensorimotor interpretation of aphasia that is inadequate because it accounts for no relation whatever between speech and thought. Nevertheless, in succession, Kussmaul (1876), Lichtheim (1885), and Grasset (1907) attempted to adjoin to the various image centers a "superior" center, covering them all: the center of concept formation, or the ideation center.

In fact, it was the abandonment of images that led to a new interpretation of aphasia. For Bergson (1911), it was "meaning above all that guides us in the reconstitution of forms and sounds," so that speech cannot then be simply a mechanical succession of sensory and motor images, and aphasia thus becomes a disturbance in the realization of thought.

Yet for Pierre Marie (1906) there existed only the aphasia described by Wernicke, in which the disturbance in comprehension is brought about solely by "intellectual impairment which must dominate the doctrine of aphasia." Indications of such impairment would be gaps in professional knowledge and in conventional or descriptive mimicry, difficulty with calculation and with understanding spoken language. It should be noted that certain disturbances that Marie cited as proofs (such as apraxia and acalculia) have now been recognized as distinctly separate from aphasia, as the lesion responsible for aphasia extends into other functional cerebral zones. Marie's thesis did have the merit of giving aphasia a unitary status, and above all, the merit of putting the disorder back into the framework of cognitive functions; but by confusing thought and speech, it denied to speech all autonomy and all specificity.

Jackson (1864–1893), noting the marked contrast between aphasics' conservation of automatic aspects of speech side by side with alterations in its "voluntary" aspects, showed that aphasia is characterized by loss of the propositional use of words, that is, of the links that the patient can forge between words to create a proposition. Further, there is no difference between external speech and internal speech, which represent the expressive aspect and the audiphonatory aspect of thought. Jackson's distinction between automatic and voluntary aspects of perception led him to describe propositions of perception as the basis for organization of the perceptive whole. Thought is made up of reciprocal exchanges between two aspects in which visual representations help to make precise word meanings in a proposition constructed by the subject and in which speech selects perceived or evoked images. Jackson, within the logic of his system, described three forms of aphasia, one concerning the auditory-articulatory processes of verbalization, the second the retino-ocular processes of representation, the third being a combination of the two preceding forms.

Head (1926) synthesized this double aspect in Jackson's idea of thought into the "symbolic function." A word or a mental image has ceased to be the single trace of an anterior perception and has become a symbol. Aphasia represents a disorder in symbolic formulation; thus, disturbances are found in the areas of behavior in which a symbol, verbal or otherwise, is an intermediary between the conception and the execution of the act. Thus, when the aphasic cannot reproduce the gestures of the examiner (for the act, in order to be correctly reversed, would need to be evoked and translated into a verbal formulation), it is possible that this is caused by a specific disorder in the organization of the gesture: apraxia. And paradoxically, of the four aphasias described by Head, only one, nominal aphasia (difficulty in seizing the meaning of words), is truly a symbolic function disorder. Nevertheless, Head's interpretation is of capital importance from two standpoints: Speech functions as the link between conception and oral expression, making possible, according to Ombredanne's (1951) felicitous formula, the explicit elaboration of thought. This mediating function in turn depends on the use of the symbolic function of speech, or, as we would now say, of signs.

Today, the theoretical problems raised by aphasia have shifted. Aphasia has become a field for the application of linguistic theories rather than theories of thought. The sign has replaced the image, and signification has replaced representation.

It no longer seems possible to treat the different forms of aphasia as the diverse consequences of a disorder in a univocal and general "function." Aphasia can be defined as a defect of utilization of the rules permitting the encoding and decoding of a verbal message. Hence, current classifications of the aphasias attempt to define precisely which functional level of speech is impaired and to connect the disorder to a lesion in one of the physiological cerebral systems that is instrumental in speech. It is upon these criteria that Luria (1966) and Hecaen (1972), for example, sought to individualize the different forms of aphasia. One can say that reliance upon any theory of thought to explain aphasia has been abandoned.

And yet, there is no doubt that misuse of the semantic rules that organize the relations between different linguistic signs necessarily entails a disturbance of thought. Signs, linguistic or not, constitute the indispensable intermediaries of the operations of thought.

Two classes of data demonstrate this: (1) Results obtained in nonverbal intelligence tests can be normal in aphasics (Tissot, Lhermitte, and Ducarne, 1963). Likewise, analysis of the performance of patients subjected to an associative experiment (Lhermitte and Signoret, 1969) shows that the deficit in understanding depends on the degree of impairment in this operative capacity. In fact, it has not been possible to identify as specific entities the physiological systems of the brain, for a single cerebral structure can be involved in functions distinct from one another; hence, the performance of a task designed to gauge intellectual capacity varies from one aphasic to another, depending on whether or not the lesion has affected the physiological cerebral systems. (2) On the other hand, an aphasic can distort the meaning of words even when oral comprehension is apparently normal. This problem was approached (Lhermitte, Derouesne, and Lecours, 1971) by studying how aphasics classified a list of words that were semantically connected with a stimulus word, either monosemous or polysemous. The existence or absence among the classified words of semantic links with the meaning or meanings of the stimulus word made it possible to examine, in a manner both objective and dynamic, the disintegration of semantic fields. In all aphasics, these fields are disorganized, and this disorganization has little to do with deterioration of intellectual capacities. Thus, the semantic content of thought is affected apart from its operative capacities.

Piaget and Inhelder (1963) distinguished, while recognizing as complementary, two aspects of cognitive function: the operative aspect and the figurative aspect. The latter appears as a copy of the real or representation through perception, imitation, and mental image. In 1966, presenting a synthesis of their work, these authors combined in the semiotic function everything that enables the subject to imagine something—imitation, symbolic play, drawing, mental image, memories, pictures, language. Thus, along with the operative aspect, there exists a semiotic aspect of thought. It is representations that permit thought to detach itself from action and to multiply operations. Here speech plays a particularly important role, especially since its role is not limited to this representative aspect; it also provides the subject with "cognitive instruments (relation, classifications, etc.) at the service of thought" (Piaget and Inhelder, 1966). So it is understandable that the aphasic's thought would necessarily be handicapped. If one is willing to see in the notion of representation anything other than the more or less palpable evocation of a mental image, and if one is willing to admit that any meaning is, through a sign, the representation of something, then meaning must be returned to its place among other forms of representation. Study of such a phenomenon in the aphasic, which has not, to our knowledge, been undertaken, could make an important contribution to this problem.

REFERENCES

Bergson, H., *La perception du changement* (Oxford: Clarendon Press, 1911).

Broca, P.,"Perte de la parole, ramollissement chronique et destruction partielle du lobe antérieur gauche du cerveau," *Bull. Soc. d'Anthropologie,* 1861, pp. 235–238.

Dejérine, J., *L'Aphasie sensorielle et l'aphasie motrice* (Paris: La Presse Medicale, 1906), p. 14.

Finkelnburg, F. C., Niederrheinische Gesellschaft, Sitzung vom 21. März 1870 in Bonn, *Berlin. Klin. Wochenschr.,* 1870.

Fritsch, G., and Hitzig, E., Über die elektrische Erregbarkeit des Grosshirns, *Raymond's Archiv.* (Reicherts und Du Bois, 1870).

Grasset, J., "La fonction du langage et la localisation des centres psychiques dans le cerveau," *Rev. de Philosophie,* 1907.

Geschwind, N., "Disconnexion syndromes in animals and man," *Brain, 88:* 237–294, 585–644, 1965.

Head, H., *Aphasia and Kindred Disorders of Speech* (Cambridge: Cambridge University Press, 1926).

Hecaen, H., *Introduction à la neuropsychologie* (Paris: Larousse, 1972).

Jackson, H., *Selected Writings of John Hughlings Jackson,* ed. by J. Taylor, G. Holmes, and F. M. R. Walshe, (London: Hodder and Stoughton, 1931–1932).

Kussmaul, A., *Les troubles de la parole,* traduction par A. Rueff (Paris: 1884).

Lhermitte, F., and Signoret, J. L., "Analyse d'un apprentissage associatif. Résultats obtenus chez 42 aphasiques," *Cortex, 5:*415–439, 1969.

Lhermitte, F., Derouesne, J., and Lecours, A. R., "Contribution à l'étude des troubles sémantiques dans l'aphasie," *Revue Neurologique, 125:* 81–101, 1971.

Lichtheim, L., "Über Aphasie," *Dtsches. Arch. f. Klin. Med.,* 1885, p. 36.

Luria, A. R., *Higher cortical functions in man* (London: Tavistock, 1966).

Marie, P., "Revision de la question de l'aphasie: la troisième circonvolution frontale gauch ne joue aucum rôle spécial dans la fonction du langage, *Semaine Médicale,* 21:241–247, 1906.

———, *Travaux et mémoires* (Paris: Masson, 1926).

Meyerson, I., "Les Images" in *Nouveau Traité de Psychologie,* G. Dumas and F. Parie, (eds.) (Paris: Alcan, 1932), vol. II, pp. 540–606.

Meynert, J., "Der Bau der Grosshirnrinde," *Vierteljahresft. f. Psych.* (Leipzig: 1867).

Ombredanne, A., *L'Aphasie et l'élaboration de la pensée explicite* (Paris: Presses Universitaires de France, 1951).

Piaget, J. and Inhelder, B., *Les images mentales in Traité de Psychologie Expérimentale,* P. Fraisse et J. Piaget (Paris: Presses Universitaires de France, 1963), vol. VII, pp. 65–108.

———, *La psychologie de l'enfant* (Paris: Presses Universitaires de France, 1966).

Tissot, R., Lhermitte, F., and Ducarne, B., "Etat intellectuel des aphasiques. Essai d'une nouvelle approche à travers les épreuves perceptives et opératoires," *L'Encéphale,* 52:285–320, 1963.

Trousseau, A., "De l'aphasie, maladie décrite récemment sous le nom impropre d'aphémie," *Gaz des Hôp.,* 1864, p. 37.

Wernicke, C., *Der aphasische Symptomen Komplex* (Breslau: Cohn & Weigert, 1874).

Henri Ey

17

Hughlings Jackson's Fundamental Principles Applied to Psychiatry[1]

In the monograph[2] that I published with J. Rouart in 1938, which was designed to prepare a neo-Jacksonian orientation for psychiatry, we were able to reduce the work of Hughlings Jackson to four ideas: evolution of the nervous functions, hierarchy of functions, the negative and positive symptoms of dissolution, and the distinction between local and uniform dissolution in neurology and psychiatry. They were essential for us, but had not been made sufficiently explicit by the illustrious neurologist and were even less understood by those for whom they were intended. I recapitulate them here.

EVOLUTION OF THE NERVOUS FUNCTIONS

It is his teacher, Laycock, but also Charles Bell, Baillarger, Anstie, and Ribot, whom Hughlings Jackson (in his first "Croonian Lecture") claims as his kindred in thought. And, of course, it is from the philosophy of Herbert Spencer that he borrows his own model of the evolution and dissolution of nervous functions.

It is the idea of evolution, that is to say, the introduction of the time factor into the nervous system and the organization of its functions, that constitutes the basic idea that inspired him to read Herbert Spencer and Charles Darwin.

---

1. Excerpts from Ey, H., *Des idées de H. Jackson à un modèle Organo-Dynamique de la Psychiatrie.* (Toulouse: Privat, in press).

2. Ey H., and Rouart, J., *Essai d'application des principes de H. Jackson à la conception dynamique de la Neuro-Psychiatrie.* (Paris: Doin, 1938).

At the end of the eighteenth century and the beginning of the nineteenth century, biology was born of the introduction of temporality into the organization of living beings. The history of natural history and, finally, of biology has, of course, been the constant object of speculation of every philosopher, physicist, chemist, alchemist, zoologist, botanist, and naturalist even before the organization of living beings was prescribed and circumscribed by the biologists. This general sense of a universal mathesis is discovered in the speculations of the great philosophers of the classic age (Descartes, Leibnitz, Kant), who after the scholars of the Renaissance (Aldrovandi, Cardan, Ambroise Paré, Harvey, Fernel), quite naturally dreamed with Newton and Hobbes of a general logic of beings. Natural history as biology begins only with the separation, in the order of creation, of living species. If, as is said, we owe to Jonston the first *Natural History of the Quadrupeds* (1657), it is obviously not to him alone that we must attribute a discovery that was not a pulverization of forms, but that required the observation and experimentation necessary to the knowledge of the evolution of species and of each of their individual examples.

These reflections suffice to express what our own reflections owe to the two most forceful accounts of natural history produced in recent years in France by an "archaeology of knowledge" and a genealogy of ideas that, in the eighteenth and nineteenth centuries, founded biology. In fact, in *Les Mots et Les Choses* by Michel Foucault, 1966 (Classer p. 140 and p. 176, and Cuvier pp. 275–292) and in *La Logique du Vivant* by Fr. Jacob (1972) are brought to light the intertwined ontological and gnoseological roots from which the tree of life springs. I think that no reading of Buffon, Cuvier, Lamarck, or Darwin will henceforth be possible without its being refracted in the clarity and profundity of this logic of the organization of the living that calls for the archaeology of its knowledge.

Biology thus was constituted as the natural history of living beings only in taking possession of its object: living bodies. It separated itself from a cosmology that encompasses the classification of the visible forms of all beings. The theory of generalized evolution—which consists in substituting for an arbitrary and providential creation a progressive and spontaneous creation, leaving indefinitely open the solution of the problem of the origin and the end of nature in general and man in particular—is not the one that directly interested the naturalists of the eighteenth century or the biologist of the nineteenth century.

Yet, the very idea of an organization of the living being necessarily implies that its constitution, like its reproduction, is subject to a dialectic of the one and the multiple, of the like and the different and subject to it in the very proportion to which life appears in its true dimension, which is that of time. The idea of evolution thus carries in it this construction inherent in that which opposes continuity: the constancy of the being in its being—and of change.

No life of any living being is founded without this original creation of each organism, which springs from the conjunction of the possible determined by its plan of genetic organization and the possible offered by the milieu. The genetic and epigenetic points of view are not opposed, but complementary.

For Spencer, evolution is a modality of progressive complexity of living organisms that records the order of species in the chronological table of a natural history whose periods are superimposed in the geological strata. Inspired more by Newton or Laplace than by Leibnitz or Hegel, he refers unceasingly to this mechanical model of universal evolution, governed by the fundamental principle of "an integration of matter and concomitant dissipation of motion, during which the matter passes from an indefinite, incoherent homogeneity to a definite, coherent heterogeneity." But this "coherence" and this "incoherence" are reversible, depending only upon the consequences of the conservation of force. However, upon this machinery to which the Spencerian conception of evolution is too often reduced there is superimposed, in connection with the passage from the homogeneous to the heterogeneous, a less mechanical conception that, while borrowing its mechanical elements from the sensationism of Hume, constantly calls upon the operational or functional concepts of integration.

And the evolutionism of Hughlings Jackson—even if it often seems attached to the conception of a sort of rational mechanics—and of Herbert Spencer reflects still more profoundly the idea of a dynamism that unifies the hierarchy of forms. In this Jackson became the pioneer of the application of the principles of biology to neurobiology. What constitutes the axis of his thought is the idea of becoming, by which the organization of an organism is constituted and directed, integrating at superior levels what is specifically and more soundly integrated at inferior levels. Such is the most profound meaning of the fundamental intuition of Jackson's ideas on functional metamorphoses:[3] the central nervous system is the place where time inscribes its requirement, that of becoming, of "creative evolution."

---

3. An expression clarified by W. Riese in *Principles of Neurology in the Light of History and Their Present Use* (New York: Nervous and Mental Disease Monographs, 1950).

HIERARCHY OF FUNCTIONS

For the image fixed in its mechanical constancy of a visible structure "seen" only in the simultaneity of its forms and movements, the eighteenth century substituted that of an organization that entails order and the subordination of the parts to the whole. For, as we have just seen, the introduction of time is not only equivalent to watching over the unfolding of the successive phases of forms and movements, but of assigning them a plan of organization (a strategy). This notion of a functional hierarchy in the organization of the functions of the nervous system, so far as they are integrated, was quite naturally to be made the keystone of Jackson's system of the "nervous system." But by limiting himself too strictly to a "spatial hierarchy," copied from that of the medullary segments, he risked missing the point of the functional hierarchy of the levels of integration of the relational life, which is organized not only *in*, but also *by* the central nervous system; he missed dynamism (the internal and constant evolution of the living brain) by limiting himself to a superimposition of mechanical reflex devices.

Let us not forget that when Jackson was developing an architectonic model of neuropsychic organization, neurophysiology was dominated (as it still is today) by the idea that the unit of the nervous system is the reflex[4]—the automatic reflection of movement upon its stimulus in such a way that its configuration appears as a simple geometrical-mechanical structure. Indeed, Descartes, Thomas Willis, and Baglivi, and then Marshall Hall (1831) proposed to make the reflex arc the essential structure of the central nervous system. Nothing seems to correspond better to the idea of autonomous and superimposed segments of the nervous system (whose medulla offers the most obvious morphology), in which, at each level, there is set in motion (according to a simple linking of response to its stimulus) the same associative preformed apparatus (conditioned reflex).

So far as the autonomy of segments is concerned, comparative anatomy provides the phylogenetic model of the segmentary structure of worms or insects formed of superimposed rings, isolable and perdurable, in their automatic activity after the cutting of the linear chain. The consideration of decapitated animals (cf. the chapter that Can-

---

4. Cf. J. Soury, *Le Système Nerveux Central.* Carre et Naud, 1899, 2 vol., G. Canguilhem, *La Formation du Concept de Réflexe aux XVIIème et XVIIIème siècles.* Paris, P.U.F., 1955; M. Merleau-Ponty, *Structure du Comportement* (pp. 1–64), Paris, Gallimard, 1942; W. Blasius, "Zur Geschichte der Reflexlehre unter besonderer Würdigung des Beitrages von Paul Hoffmann," (*Deutsche Z.f. Nervenheil.* 1965, *186*:475–495).

guilhem devotes to this subject) had already long interested the scholars of the eighteenth century. (Blumenbach, it seems, already counted 232 theories on the automatic movement of these animal fragments!) The frog became the hero and the first victim of sectioning experiments (Fulton); but vipers, salamanders, and turtles furnished the physiologists of this period with abundant material for observation and experimentation on the autonomy of the automatic movements of these segmented organisms. The works of J. A. Unzer (1771), G. Proscheska (1784), and S. Holes (1750) quite naturally prepared the way for neurophysiology to describe with precision the reflexes of the frog with isolated medulla or of the decapitated dog. Whence Pflüger's famous laws of the reflexes (1853), which state precisely the characteristics of localization, of the radiation of movements, which manifest by their autonomy, their regularity, and their absence of finality that their capacity to function is contained in the superimposed segments of the medulla.[5]

The idea of a spatial hierarchy of the sensorimotor centers was thus in the minds of most of the anatomists, physiologists, and pathologists of the nervous system. But this spatial and mechanical (Magoun was to call it "geleological") conception hardly satisfied Jackson, who refused to identify strictly the seat of the lesion, functional center, and anatomical location.

He had accepted and long since developed the idea that the evolution of the functions of the nervous system constitutes an "ascending development," characterized by the passage from the most organized (that is to say, the most closely connected and fixed) lower to the less stably organized higher centers (first "Croonian Lecture"). But Jackson also untiringly repeated that—evolution being a simple passage from the simplest to the most complex, between the inferior centers and the centers of the "highest level"—there was only a sort of graduation in this complexity,[6] to the point of considering the

---

5. I set forth in my *Traité des Hallucination* (Paris: Masson, 1973) the ideas of Charles Sherrington, who submitted the Jacksonian model of the integration of the central nervous system to the most subtle experimental scrutiny (pp. 1087–1093). I also added to this an exposition on the Pavlovian reflex doctrine and cybernetics (pp. 1094–1099).

6. He says in this first "Croonian Lecture" that there is no contradiction in speaking of centers as being at the same time most complex and least organized. The fact is that organization exists even in the simple centers and is a constant, whereas complexity is only a variable.

This idea, so thoroughly developed in all Jackson's works, is expressed for the first time with great precision of explanation in his memoir of 1881: "On Some Implications of Dissolution of the Nervous System," (*Selected Writings of John Hughlings Jackson*, ed. by James Taylor, Gordon Holmes, and F. M. R.

higher centers to be of the same nature (the same structuring of nervous elements and the same functional sensorimotor reflex value). Still, while indicating that evolution is a passage from the most automatic to the most voluntary,[7] Jackson nevertheless introduced a new and fundamental dimension into the pyramidal organization of the nervous system. The notion of organization in general, so closely linked to the idea of evolution, compelled him to join to the idea of superimposition that of hierarchy, and to the idea of meshing that of integration. For Jackson, that which is superimposed in space is that which succeeds in time, and that which is inferior because of being more fixed is subordinate to what is superior because of being more contingent. Such is the teleology implied in the hierarchy of nervous functions: The inferior or instrumental functions at the control of the highest level, building up like words into syntax,[8] means to an end. In other words, in spite of the apparent mechanicalism, Jackson could propose a model of graded structuring of the central nervous system that was an ontogenesis of the autonomy of relational life, rather than a model of the architecture of the spinal column. And concerning the "highest level," Max Levin (1961) points out that Jackson attributed to it the function of the coordination of impressions and movements ("vivid images," "faint images"); the "highest level" (more complex and less organized) is thus the equivalent of a synthesis, less automatic than that "vigilance" that Head was to grant to the simplest reflex arc. Thus, it is not in the complexity, but in the activity of the function of integration that we find the principle of functional hierarchy. To be sure, Russel Brain (1958) rightly pointed out that there are no fundamentally different levels in integration, inasmuch as the latter, at all levels, effects essentially a sensorimotor coordination. But what must define the "highest level" is, as Jackson said, its contingency, its freedom. For the automatic and the voluntary are the logical instances of functional hierarchy, whose morphology, the visible and invisible arrangements of the nervous system, constitutes only the

---

Walshe (London: Hodder and Stoughton, 1931–32) vol. 2, pp. 29–44). It seems to me that the correct interpretation of this very abstract passage from Jackson's writings (cf. 41–44) enables us to understand better how, in fact the lower centers (medulla, rhombencephalon) represent directly the parts of the body, the middle centers are re-representative of the parts of the body entailing a double (or indirect) representation (central grey matter), and the highest centers represent the entire organism.

7. Paradoxically, this notion of the most voluntary, which gives its full meaning to the hierarchical system of nervous functions, was considered vulgar by Jackson, and he intended, without ever being able to achieve it, to abandon the idea and even suppress the term!

8. Jackson explained this idea most clearly in his studies on aphasia.

phases of the free movement of the relational life. In this respect, Jackson's ideas are most akin to those of Baillarger.

Jackson's consideration of the problem posed by the "highest level centers" was constant from 1880 on. It is quite certain that his studies on aphasia and notably on epilepsy led him to form an idea of the functioning of the centers of language and of consciousness.

As for the "centers" of language,[9] he conceived them as the support of a hierarchy of functions, rising from the most automatic to the most voluntary, from sensorimotor association to propositional expression, from exclamative language to the speech of categorical thought, as Kurt Goldstein was to call it later.[10]

The notion of the "center of consciousness" has remained the stumbling block of the Jacksonian theory of the hierarchy of functions even in the mind of Jackson. It is a question of the summit of evolution and of the hierarchy of nervous functions that constitute the "organ of mind," an expression Jackson always put in quotation marks. This "highest level," according to Jackson, is never anything but the instrument of the mind and does not constitute the mind. It is precisely there that his "parallelism" encounters its own contradiction and that, as commentators have pointed out (Riese, Schlesinger, Gooddy, Walshe, etc.), he has slipped from the idealistic dualism of the relation of mind (consciousness) to matter (brain), into a gestaltist "isomorphism," as Köhler pointed out.

Strict observation of facts enabled Jackson to escape the contradictions of the system of "concomitance" of mind and brain. For by substituting a plan of organization of the nervous system that is ascending, he caused the parallels to converge; more exactly, he transformed them into the arrow of an evolution that implies passage from the automatic to the voluntary, in order to make possible the "autorealization of the organism beyond its elementary aims," as Goldstein was to say. The idea of a "Gestalt" as the very configuration of every act of consciousness is indicated in the second text of 1887, "Remarks on Evolution and Dissolution,"[11] in which he endeavors to close the

---

9. Cf. "Speech Affections from Brain Diseases" (1879–1880) in *Selected Writings*, vol. 2, pp. 171–204), especially pp. 198–204, and "Words and Other Symbols in Mentation" (1893), in *Selected Writings*, vol. 2, pp. 205–212.

10. All the great works on language pathology in relation to brain pathology (Pick, Head, Goldstein, Cassirer, Luria, etc.) are inspired directly by the Jacksonian notion of evolution and hierarchy of functions that compose discursive communication. Reference to it is found again in contemporary psycho-neuro-linguistic studies (Hecaen, Lhermitte, particularly), when they resort to the functional stratification of the levels, structures and uses of language (de Saussure, Jacobson, Chomsky, etc.).

11. *Selected Writings*, vol. II, pp. 92–97.

gap that seems to separate consciousness from its object, form from its content, and in which he insists upon the fact that the functions (will, memory, reason, emotion) are artificially separated. In this text, Jackson makes it definite that the "anatomical substrata" of subject consciousness are more perfectly organized than the "anatomical substrata" of object consciousness. The activity of consciousness at its highest level characterizes that very integration of the two parallels that the principle of concomitance would keep eternally apart. For Jackson discovered that the brain *contains*[12] the "dream of the action," so that while continuing to affirm (like Henri Bergson in "Matiére et Mémoire") that it is only the instrument of thought (conscious mind), by the very notion of integration at the "highest level" he considers it as the organizer, the subject and the author of its own organization.[13]

DISSOLUTION, ITS NEGATIVE AND POSITIVE SYMPTOMS

This dynamism that confers its meaning upon symptoms is that of "subsisting instances" of what the lesion leaves intact. The latter can be of the destructive type (*destroying lesion*) or of the discharge type (*discharging lesion*). In both cases there are negative effects, a suppression or disorder of the nerve centers at whatever level, and positive effects that give evidence of the subjacent activity at the functional level affected, or of the still healthy juxtaposed parts that surround the altered functional zone and are more or less connected with it. In the lecture that Hughlings Jackson delivered on December 8,

---

12. When he points out (for example in 1884 in the Third "Croonian Lecture" *Selected Writings*, vol. 2, p. 67) that the lowest centers are not only "reservoirs of images," but "resisting positions," he is, in fact, contemplating integration in its most "reflex" or "automatic" form, but it is also a function of control or inhibition that he attributes to the higher centers, as he insists at length in his discussion before the Neurological Society in 1888 (in referring to his "Croonian Lectures."

13. Walther Riese stressed the dynamic, evolving, unfolding, and open character of the system represented by the psychic whole.

> The hierarchy of nervous function should therefore not be conceived as a fixed and rigid one-way dominance exerted by the higher levels, but rather as a mobile control exerted by one level over the others, according to circumstances and susceptible of being reversed under new conditions. No level seems to be in possession of a permanent chief position and the whole system seems to be built on the model of the equality and the reciprocity of the parts (i.e., of a republic of mature citizens). [*Principles of Neurology*, (Baltimore: Williams and Wilkins, 1950), 32].

1897 to the Neurological Society,[14] he presents as examples of his interpretation of dissolution various nervous affections, particularly epilepsy in its different convulsive and psychical aspects.[15]

If in paralysis the destructive effect of the lesion on motor function is obvious, the negative cause of "epileptic discharges" is less so. It is essentially a question of a gross disorder (to translate "coarse change") of the arrangements of the motor centers. Tonic and clonic movements manifest the loss of coordination constituting their negative condition; the effect of the lesion, and their disharmony characterizes the hyperactivity of functional elements freed from the normally inhibiting action (control) of their activity.

We discover here, with Jackson, the articulation (one might say the dialectic) of the negative and the positive in the pathogenesis and symptomatology of nervous disorders. If, in fact, pathogenesis is not mechanical, even at this level of convulsive movements, the symptom is not the direct effect of the lesion. The visible and manifest symptom (a word mispronounced or uttered instead of another, trembling instead of movement firmly set upon its course, or an imposed regularity upon the tonus of violent rhythms), manifests the latency[16] of the fundamental disturbance, which is the disorganization of a functional system of a certain level of integration. So, even at the most "neurological" level, the symptoms are clinically positive, but they are also necessarily negative in revealing the disorder that engenders them. Symptomatology is, in its manifestation, relatively independent of the negative trouble ("organo-clinical distance," let us say), while pathogenically it is always dependent upon it.

In this connection, it is to the principle formulated by F. E. Anstie (in his book *Stimulants and Narcotics*) that Hughlings Jackson re-

---

14. *Selected Writings*, vol. 2, pp. 422–443.

15. Besides the texts reproduced in our 1938 monograph, I likewise recommend almost all of the first volume of the *Selected Writings*, especially pp. 135–160 of the work "*Epilepsy and After-Effects of Discharges,*" pp. 178–190 in the memoir of the same year entitled "On the Scientific and Empirical Investigation of Epilepsy" (particularly the passage on pp. 178–190 and in vol. 2, pp. 76–118), and "Remarks on Evolution and Dissolution of the Nervous System," a memoir that appeared in the *Journal of Mental Science* in April, 1887.

16. One might say that "subjacency" of the fundamental disturbance, to emphasize the fact that the latter, while determining the positive manifestation (being the cause of this effect), remains less directly visible to the clinician's eye and less perceptible to the consciousness of the patient himself. For, in the fact, the negative alteration is a disappearance necessary to the appearance of the symptom," which is, like the dream, for the observer or the dreamer himself, but only to their respective reflection, a phenomenon of sleep.

fers.[17] This principle[18] of the "loss of control" of the higher centers, permitting overactivity of the inferior functions, has since 1874 (British Medical Journal) been applied by Hughlings Jackson at the level of movements, sensations, or disturbances of language as well as at the level of "insanities" and to the epileptic "discharging lesion."[19] He extended the applications of this principle even into minute analyses of epileptic, choreic, aphasic, and Parkinsonian syndromes.

It is almost always to the pathogenesis of the "insanities" (mental diseases) that Jackson, and all the authors with whom he agreed, apply this notion of escape from control in the field of psychiatry rather than in that of neurology. Neurological disturbances, being of a lower level and a more "local" structure, lend themselves to analysis with greater difficulty.

The sphere of psychiatry constitutes the field of cerebral pathology in which is most manifestly verified the theory of the dissolution of nervous functions and of its double negative and positive effect. When Jackson refers to it explicitly,[20] his descriptions and reflections bear witness to his preoccupation with showing how the putting out of action of the superior levels exalts the automatism of the inferior levels. It is in this perspective that he read in his first "Croonian Lecture"[21] these sentences:

> I submit that disease only produces negative mental symptoms answering to the dissolution, and that all elaborate positive mental symptoms (illusions, hallucinations, delusions, and extravagant conduct) are the outcome of activity of nervous elements untouched by any pathological process. . . . The most absurd mentation and the most extravagant actions in insane people are the survivals of their fittest states.

---

17. *Selected Writings*, vol. 1, p. 123 (note), p. 176 (note), p. 226 (note), and vol. 2, pp. 6 and 8, and especially the "Croonian Lectures," and "Factors of Insanities."

18. Anstie wrote notably: "The apparent exaltation of certain faculties should be described as arising from the suppression of their control rather than from a positive stimulation of these faculties." I should have placed this sentence as an epigraph to my *Traité des Hallucinations,* and more particularly to the chapter that (like Anstie) I devoted to the hallucinogens.

19. On the subject of this crucial point, the whole work entitled "Some Implications of Dissolution," 1882 (*Selected Writings,* vol. 2, pp. 29–44), should be read and meditated upon. It is in this article (one of the most profound that he wrote) that, in the note to p. 39 he says: "The correct statement of my opinions would be that 'the theory of discharges' is *not* the pathology of epilepsies."

20. *Selected Writings*, vol. 2, pp. 6–9, 25–28, 405–420, 441, et passim.

21. Ibid., pp. 46–47.

His illusions, etc., are not caused by the disease, but are the outcome of activity of what is left of him [of what disease has spared], of all there then is of him; his illusions, etc., are his mind.

When Bleuler, inspired by the psychodynamic studies of Freud and Jung, says that almost all the "symptomatology of schizophrenia is secondary in relation to the primary process," Jacksonian intuition should appear as the founder of all psychopathology. The fact is that, just as a neurological syndrome (e.g., chorea, aphasia) can be explained only by a thorough knowledge of the normal physiology of the levels of movement or linguistic operations, in psychiatry mental disease appears as a "liberation"[22] of the "lower level of activity."

As Jackson so often said, the idea of evolution and the idea of dissolution of the nervous structure are organized around the more or less automatic. So the notion of automatism involves at the same time the positive and negative component of nervous pathology.[23] We shall see that this nervous pathology, particularly cerebral pathology, cannot be visualized on the same model. For the moment it is important to emphasize that for Jackson automatic activity constitutes the positive component. Convulsions, like impulsions, paraphasic speech, agnosia, apraxia, delirium, and hallucinations, represent the living and healthy *reaction* to the pathological disturbance, an effort to reestablish homeostasis. But what has been too often forgotten is that psychological automatism is pathological only when it results from a negative condition. When it is a question of a spasm or convulsion, to say that it is a phenomenon of nervous discharge is to imply that this discharge is the product of a mechanical or electrical excitation of nervous elements, which constitutes a heterogeneous pathological positivity (a neoproduction). But we know well that contemporary neurophysiology and neuropathology (since Jackson) considers the "discharging phenomenon" as the effect of a negative disturbance; all the more reason when it is a question of a mental disease, where the organo-clinical distance is greatest and where the positive symptomatology is richest, even to the point of masking the negative condition on which the positivity of the psychopathological symptoms depends. So that this negativity is denied by the partisans of a

---

22. The term is sometimes employed, for instance in the Memoir of 1881 on the dissolution and the epileptic states (*Selected Writings*, vol. 2, p. 19), particularly in the sense of liberation of energy, but is more often replaced by "survival of the fittest." *Unleashing* in English, *entbinden* in German, *debinden* in French may be the most fitting translation of Jackson's thought for the manifestation of pathological activity that due to the defect of high level activity is deprived of control.

23. Cf. my *Traité des Hallucinations*, pp. 905, 954, 1254, et passim.

pure psychogenesis (without negative process) of mental diseases.[24]

And by this reflection we go back to what we have already said about the Jacksonian intuition of evolution. The automatism that the negative pathogenic condition unleashes is necessarily the unconscious. Freud had not yet spoken when Jackson was writing, and one would not be able to reproach him for not seeing in the positivity of liberated automatisms the instinctive or libidinal forces he integrated into the remaining positivity.

Thus, complementary analysis, the dialectic of the negative and the positive, must be considered as the common foundation of neurological and psychiatric science.

NEUROLOGY AND PSYCHIATRY:
THE DISTINCTION BETWEEN TWO TYPES OF
LOCAL AND UNIFORM DISSOLUTION

The application of the theory of evolution and dissolution of nervous functions is reserved exclusively for the physiological "arrangement" of the nervous system, with perpetual concern not to confuse its functional hierarchy with psychical activity.[25] We have emphasized that the principle of "concomitance" was not strictly respected when it reached the "highest level" and the theory of mental disorders. So that, if one seeks in Jackson's ideas a way to differentiate the sphere of neurology from the sphere of psychiatry, one must return to the notions of "center" and "dissolution."

The notion of "highest centers" should hold our attention. For Jackson—who always speaks of them in the plural, recognizing that each of the four centers (memory, attention, movement, emotion) is a sort of abstract entity—this functional stratification ("layers of highest centers") is never considered otherwise than as an algebraic sum of homogeneous parts. In his system, the "highest level" is not merely an order composed of more and more numerous elements in which is reflected the greatest part or the totality of the body.[26]

---

24. A. de Waelhens (to cite the opinion of one of the most serious philosophers of our time), who, under the aegis of certain psychiatrists, has committed the error of opting for an exclusively psychogenetic view of the psychoses.

25. Faithful of his theory of concomitance, he affrms in his first "Lumleian Lecture" at the Royal College (1890) that there is no more a physiology of the mind than there is a psychology of the nervous system (*Selected Writings*, vol. 1, p. 417)—that, basically, the psychologist must be first a physiologist. For me, it is the reverse that is true, without losing sight of the fact that both have the same object.

26. *Selected Writings*, vol. 2, p. 400.

But in introducing the idea of a more fixed and specific integration at the inferior levels and, consequently, a more free and personal one at the superior levels in addition to that of an application of the notions of "highest level" and its dissolution to "insanities," the very principle of functional hierarchy involved that of concomitance. Therefore, the "hierarchy of the centers" assumes a *subordination* of the automatic to the voluntary. This idea is the corollary of the very idea of progressive evolution or of functional hierarchy. So that at the level of the "mental highest centers" we must consider them *in their activity*, not only as instruments of consciousness but as effecting the very integration of the organization as a whole. And thereby the very principle of a sameness of structural organization—modeled on the reflex or on cybernetic reverberations—is put in question again. It is advisable to substitute for it the far more Jacksonian idea of levels of integration, so that the "highest level," being that of global integration,[27] can only bring about their dissolution by its disintegration, itself global (uniform, said Jackson); while dissolution at subordinate levels can bring about only a partial or instrumental disintegration.

Whence the distinction introduced by Jackson between *uniform* (or global) *disolution* and *local* (or partial) *dissolution*.

In uniform dissolution, Jackson tells us,[28] the evolution of the nervous system is reversed, so that there is a general reduction of activity; though the inferior centers are more resistant than the middle ones, and the process takes place according to a "compound order." In local dissolution, the reversal of evolution does not involve the whole of the nervous system, but only a part. This dissolution may be "local," with reference either to depth or to a certain extent.

It is almost impossible, by reason of the number and prolixity of his writings, even the "selected" ones, to follow the meanders of Jackson's thought on this notion of local (or partial) dissolution of the "highest centers." Let us be content to note that, if one believes several of his analyses of it,[29] uniform dissolutions entail a much greater positive part ("internal evolution") than that of the local dissolutions ("compensation") studied especially in connection with paralyses or

---

27. "But we have highest centers made up of *universally* representing units. . . . In general the anatomical substrata of subject consciousness are centers of universal coordination, or, as we said, they are unifying cr synthesizing centers," he writes in one of his most profound works (*"Remarks on Evolution and Dissolution,"* 1887), completing those published the same year in the *Journal of Mental Science.*

28. First "Croonian Lecture," *Selected Writings,* vol. 2, p. 47.

29. E.g., *Selected Writings,* vol. 2, pp. 45–47.

convulsions[30]; also, as is the case for disturbance of language, local dissolutions constitute a sort of insubordination, as Jackson notes, for example, in his Memoir on "Speech Affections from Brain Disease."[31]

Moreover, when he undertakes in the first "Croonian Lecture" to give illustrations of the two modalities (uniform or local) or dissolution, he applies his concept of dissolution (referring almost exclusively to local dissolutions) only to progressive muscular atrophy, hemiphelia, *paralysis agitans,* epileptic seizures, chorea, and aphasia. On the other hand, as soon as he speaks of dissolutions of the "highest level," he refers to cases of mental diseases ("insanities"). Doubtless, he explains, there exists between the two groups only a difference of localization; doubtless, he admits, there is a problem posed by the comparison of progressive muscular atrophy and mental disease, but doubtless, he maintains, there exist local dissolutions of the "highest centers," and he continues to affirm the homogeneity of the reflex structures of all the nerve centers. But pathology (dissolution) at the "highest level" is incompatible with the idea of local dissolution. On almost every page of his writings (and more especially in connection with epileptic convulsions and confusions), he treats as equivalent the terms uniform dissolution and mental disease; as far as the latter is the effect, the former is the cause of an alteration of the "highest level," the one where the relations of brain and mind coincide.

For him, nerve pathology, like the functional hierarchy of the nerve centers, was one. From the viewpoint of the general principles of the evolution and dissolution of the different levels, one finds again the same schema: integration of the less and less automatic functions and dissolution of the more and more automatic ones. But at the "climax" of higher activity at the level at once the most complex, the most voluntary, the freest, the most conscious also, it is not—to go back to his comparison of the hierarchy of movement—through sending more soldiers to defend the whole territory that this territory (this organism) will be well defended. The idea of hierarchy implies not only that of a superimposition (or progressive addition) of units, but also that of subordination of the parts to the whole. So that the "highest level" is not a localized or localizable center, and its dissolution affects its own totalizing organization (the "topmost layers" and not the "highest centers"). Not being a "localizer," as Jackson says,[32] he was quite right not to wish to be so at this level; but not being a "universalizer," he owed it to himself not to be so to the point of not

30. Ibid., vol. 1, pp. 436–438, and vol. 2, pp. 35–40.

31. Ibid., vol. 2, pp. 185 (note).

32. Ibid., vol. 2, p. 35.

distinguishing more clearly between uniform dissolutions and local dissolutions.[33] For that it was necessary to make still clearer the subordination of centers (the "local" dissolution of which leads, e.g., to hemiplegia, convulsive epilepsy) in relation to the superior level of integration, which, too, is susceptible in the generative process of mental disease to uniform or global dissolution.

In treating the "insanities" as the result of a uniform dissolution (negative) liberating a psychological automatism (unconscious), Jackson provided broad access to a solution of the problem of the relations of neurology (the pathology of local dissolutions, centers and systems inferior to the "highest level") to psychiatry (the pathology of uniform dissolutions of the "highest level"). However, he did not perceive clearly enough the importance of this distinction on the theoretical plan, whereas all his studies on epileptic convulsions, paralyses, chorea, etc., on one hand, and postepileptic confusion and the various degrees of "insanities" on the other hand were nevertheless conducted by him in this perspective.

The greatest reason for this "blind spot" is obviously his postulate of parallelist "concomitance"; but more concretely, more "phenomenologically," it is that in order to speak of a dissolution of the "highest level," it is necessary to form an idea of the consciousness that this "highest level" constitutes. It would not be sufficient for him to speak of it as a state "coinciding with higher nervous activity" without saying anything more about it. Still, his studies on the different levels of the state of consciousness ought to have led him to challenge the principle of concomitance. He would then have had to admit that dissolutions of the "highest level" are the province of psychiatry, and local dissolutions are the province of neurology. For there is a fundamental distinction to be made between instrumental function and consciousness, but it is not what separates the nervous system and the "psychism"; it is what separates the integrated (or instrumental) functions from the integrating structures of the conscious being.

Such were the ideas or principles of Hughlings Jackson that had attracted my attention and my interpretation some forty years ago. It is these first intuitions and their elaboration pursued unceasingly since then that I should like to revive in presenting them anew.

---

33. Basically, his whole theoretical system, so rich and fertile for the analysis of the process of dissolution in general, is out of plumb in attempting to separate more the "nervous state" from the mental state than uniform dissolutions of the organization of the "highest level" from local dissolutions of the instrumental functions of the functional levels subject to the control of the "highest level" (organ of mind).

It is obvious that I have not abided by the letter of the great neurologist's conception. Far from it. To apply it to psychiatry without running the risk of "neurologizing" it, I had to rethink the concepts of evolution, dissolution, higher mental activity, local and uniform dissolution, etc. Consequently, it was necessary to exorcise the Jacksonian system of the principle of concomitance, so that the sphere of liberation (in the common sense of insubordination) and of an emancipation from psychological automatism (Janet) and of the unconscious (Freud), in other words, the sphere of psychopathology, should be understood by us as a pathology of freedom lost when the organization of the conscious being is dissolved. Such is, in fact, the meaning of the *natural history of insanity* that, with Jackson and, later, Freud, we have drawn from biological sources.

REFERENCES

Evans, Ph., "Henri Ey's Concepts of the Organization of Consciousness and Its Désorganization. An extension of Jacksonian theory." *Brain, 95:* 413–440, 1972.

Ey, H., *Des Idées de Jackson à un modèle Organo-Dynamique de la Psychiatrie* (Toulouse: Privat, in press).

——, *Traité des Hallucinations* (Paris: Masson, 1973), pp. 1070–1342.

——, *La Conscience*. Ière éd. 1963, 2ème éd. 1968 (Presses Universitaires de France, Paris).

Ey, H., and Rouart, J., *Essai d'Application des Principes de H. Jackson à la Conception Dynamique de la Neuro-Psychiatrie* (Paris: Doin, 1938).

Jackson, H. H., *Selected Writings of John Hughlings Jackson*. Edited by James Taylor, Gordon Holmes, and F. M. R. Walshe (London: Hodder & Stoughton, 1931–32), 2 vols.

Riese, W., "Hughlings Jackson's Doctrine of Consciousness," *J. Nerv. and Ment. Dis., 120:*330–337, 1954.

Straus, E. W., Nathan, M., and Ey, H., *Psychiatry and Philosophy* (New York: Springer, 1969), pp. 111–161.

William Gooddy

18

The Major and Minor Hemispheres
of the Human Brain

*It is to the credit of human intelligence and creativeness
to have conceived a doctrine as a mighty instrument for the
discovery of natural phenomena and yet borrowed the first
principle of this doctrine not from facts, which we worship
too much, but from a scheme or design of our own which
we underestimate too much. . . . Our first concern should
be to answer the question: which natural phenomena are
susceptible to localization and which have to be excluded
from it?*

—Walther Riese, *Principles of Neurology*

In that masterpiece of neurological philosophy, *Principles of Neurology,* which Dr. Walther Riese published in 1950, we find in the chapter "Lateral Cerebral Dominance" the statement:. "Any lesion disturbing cerebral mechanisms must be interpreted *in the light of time."*
This stimulating theme has provided a text upon which to base a
theory of space-time awareness derived from direct clinical observation of neurological cases in the field of the higher cerebral functions,
where no animal other than man can demonstrate and describe symptoms and signs.

Inside the skull lies the brain, a single organ with a double structure, each half a mirror-image of the other. We know from clinical
and pathological observation (the pyramidal tract and its decussation
were probably first described by Misticelli in 1709, the same year as
Berkeley's "A New Theory of Vision") that if either hemisphere is
damaged, we shall find an impaired function on the opposite side of

220

the body (e.g., hemianopia, and motor and sensory hemiplegia). But as practical clinicians, we have also observed from repeated findings in our patients that there are special, extra vulnerabilities of function in addition to hemiplegia, in direct relation to the side of the brain that is damaged. These disorders are commonly described as *aphasia, agnosia,* and *apraxia.*

We are now in the realms of cerebral "dominance" and of the related subject "handedness." These concepts are closely related in the neurologist's mind with matters of language and aphasia. The correlation of language disturbance with lesions of one hemisphere rather than the other was first made when Brocca in 1861 described a right-handed patient with a lesion maximum at the lower end of the motor strip on the left side of the brain. Thus, if aphasia is present in a right-handed patient, the lesion responsible will be in the left hemisphere. If the patient is left-handed, the lesion is almost certainly in the right hemisphere. There is not space here to make an exposition of the facts and underlying theories of handedness; we must accept that handedness is presumably an entirely human characteristic, and is related to language.

We have been told for many years now that what distinguishes man from hominid is his capacity to use tools; but this distinction is being lost as more examples of animal usage of tools are being found. *What truly distinguishes man from all other animals and from his own predecessors is his handedness.* We may note in what we consider the finest examples of skill that the artist and craftsman acts as a two-handed creator, with the special characteristic that he uses each hand separately at the same time. He has become a double man. This true ambidexterity is very rare, and usually is a sign of genius.

Aphasia, Agnosia, and Apraxia

In investigating the possibility of dysphasia, we use a plan of simple questioning. There are five basic questions:

1. Is the patient right-handed or left-handed, and has he always been so?
2. Is he willing and able to hear and see, and does he normally understand the language used?
3. Is he able to name a fair range of objects, chosen to suit his scholastic levels?
4. Is he able to express himself in
   (a) spoken words and other symbols?
   (b) written words and other symbols?

5. Is he able to understand
    (a) spoken words and other symbols?
    (b) written words and other symbols?

We may also test other performances allied to the language functions, mathematical calculation being one of the more important. Mathematical ideas are fundamentally related to digital knowledge, and *dyscalculia* is often associated with defective awareness and naming of individual fingers (finger-agnosia). We may also find some degree of manipulatory disturbance for chosen tasks, even when there is no obvious paralysis or sensory loss. Sequential performance in space may be lost, together with the mental imagery of actions, so that the patient may be unable to perform habitual tasks, or to "go through the motions" of tasks. To this kind of defect the term *dyspraxia* is attached. It appears to be due to a loss of the power to exteriorize activity in symbolic form, even though the underlying space-time mechanisms are undisturbed. (On the evidence of the undisturbed functioning of the space-time mechanism, patient is able to pass as normal or almost normal, unless special expressive or receptive formulations are demanded of him. He can dress, find his way about, enjoy something of hobbies or television, and even drive a car.)

These clinical facts provide the neurological evidence for using the label "dominant" for the left hemisphere of right-handed people. We now turn to the other hemisphere, the one called "minor" or "nondominant." Until recently, the brain was assumed to be "silent," it is only comparatively recently that the frontal, parietal, and temporal lobes have become accessible to clinical investigation. Far from being silent, these regions nowadays cry out for understanding. It is possible that the terms agnosia and apraxia might have had an obscuring effect upon such investigation, since they are often used in an overprecise manner, having entirely different meanings for different investigators.

Many have noted with genuine surprise that some patients—right-handed, with right-sided damage—will deny that a totally useless left arm and leg have anything wrong with them (*anosognosia*). Difficulty in dressing, or getting lost in the home or even in one room may be mentioned as oddities of behavior (sometimes causing the patient to be admitted, to a mental hospital). It is often regarded as a whimsical, almost laughable test to ask a patient to draw a clockface, a daisy, an arrow, a map. Yet the way a patient responds to this simple clinical examination for these abnormalities may give us just as much information about the site of a lesion as do the electroencephalogram, angiogram, isotope scan, or air study.

One test is of especial value in assessing whether damage has occurred to the minor hemisphere posteriorly. This test, described in *Problems of Dynamic Neurology* (Gooddy and Reinhold, 1963), also illustrates the principles of space-time. The patient is asked to draw a simple directional arrow, consisting of three lines, in various directions. If he cannot do this spontaneously, a model may be provided. The common defects are shown in Figure 1.

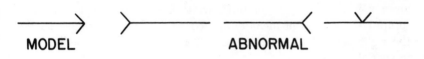

MODEL   ABNORMAL

Figure 1

What does this test signify? Why is the arrow form of such universal use in daily life? It is because of the specificity of a single direction. In a drawn arrow, we sum up our knowledge about movement through space. Movement through space implies a change with time. So when any human being makes any movement, he is performing a complicated act of space-time navigation of utmost refinement without the aid of any external map, chronometer, or compass. This most important capacity, second in importance only to the language faculty, is fundamental to daily and even momentary survival. We can now see why the arrow becomes so direction-significant. We act subconsciously as if we are schematically at the center of an ever-changing three-dimensional sphere. In practice, we schematize our position by using a map or plan, a two-dimensional form. This reduction permits us to act within a circle. We find it convenient to subdivide the circle into 360 units (degrees). In going in one chosen direction, what we do is to select that direction by rubbing out all the other 359 possible directions.

Thus, if—as seems likely—the minor hemisphere is vital to our capacity to navigate successfully in space-time, we find it easy to understand why a right-handed patient with right-sided damage should have difficulty in finding his way about, in understanding maps and plans, in constructing models that require a specific space-time set of movements, and even in dressing himself—for dressing requires first a model of the movable scheme of the person and then the relationship of a new integument, an outer skin. Therefore, it is possible that our capacity to add and subtract dimensionality (that is, to use the map or timetable as a useful representation of three- and four-dimensional space, and to use the time dimension applied to the two-dimensional map to create a successful four-dimensional journey, either from the earth to the moon or, perhaps more difficult, from a closed to an open hand is most vulnerable to lesions of the minor hemisphere.

It has been noted clinically, both by Hoff and Pötzl and by myself, that damage in the right posterior parietal region is associated with temporal disturbances. (One patient said, "I know you will laugh when I tell you, but from the moment this trouble started [an acute vascular lesion in the right postparietal region associated with a tumor] my clocks have been switched off. I can't any longer keep any notion of time.") To be brief, while this statement is not intended to apply to matters of memory and consciousness, it is suggested that the right parietal region is essential for our usage of immediate time in spatial performance.

What may we now say about the major hemisphere? We have seen ourselves, relying upon the integrity of our minor hemisphere, making our way across the large and small dimensions of the universe. We have been doing this as single individuals, without care for others, except to avoid them as obstacles. But though such a performance appears to suffice for very simple organisms, such as amoebas and bacilli and jellyfish, as soon as complexity becomes great, all animals strive to achieve signaling systems to alert other creatures to their presence, their actions, and their intentions. Insects signal, apparently, in a monotone, the significance lying in the spacing of the signal, something like our Morse code. Birds threaten and coax, and carry out formation flying as skillfully as any air force. Human beings signal that we are going to turn left or right, that we are well or ill, and so on, in the innumerable forms and usages of language.

Now these functions of language are most vulnerable to damage of the major hemisphere. With damage there, we can no longer alert anyone else to our situation or to our awareness, nor can we comprehend what others signal. So we remain confined within ourselves, though still able to carry out daily activities because we have intact use of our minor, space-time navigational hemisphere. In contrast, when the minor hemisphere is damaged, we are still able to signal, but we no longer have the space-time data on which to base accurate signaling.

To summarize the theme so far, we may say that we have two mirror-image cerebral hemispheres, which are structurally indistinguishable except insofar as they *are* mirror-images. It is possible to establish clinically that damage to the left hemisphere is associated with defects of function that are obviously different from those associated with damage to the right hemisphere. These differences enable us to make the abstraction: left hemisphere—language and signaling; right hemisphere—space-time navigation and chronometry.

THE SIGNIFICANCE OF THE CONCLUSIONS— THE ESCAPE FROM DARWINIAN TIME

The term "Darwinian time" is probably a new one, for although Darwin knew that vast expanses of time were required for the success of his theory of evolution and though he was greatly disturbed by the arrogant but inept statements of Kelvin on the brevity of the existence of the solar system, calculated on the "cooling cinder" theory, Darwin used the word "time" in an ordinary, undefined sense ("we all know what is meant by time"). There are nowadays many forms of time defined by an added adjective (mathematical time, absolute time, elapsed time, personal time, and so on), so the adjective Darwinian may be justified to signify the gradual process by which the evolution of species and of life has taken place.

> Nothing impresses the mind with the vast duration of time, according to our ideas of time, more forcibly than the conviction thus gained that subaerial agencies with apparently so little power, and which seem to work so slowly, have produced great results. [Darwin, *The Origin of Species*]

To express such ideas of evolution in modern terms, we may say that the maintenance of flexibility towards the future (inherent in the mechanism of genetics) almost always demands great durations, in order that minute structural or functional variations may accumulate and become effective. The spectacular mutation is comparatively uncommon, though this ratio may not always be maintained if radiation goes unchecked.

We must see that if some means of significantly increasing functional achievement could be devised without having to wait for anatomical changes requiring many millions of human years, a species could make great advances in a fraction of the time required by processes termed "natural." This form of achievement would be in a sudden marked advance along the time-scale of living matter. Thus, some existing forms would establish significant change in hundred-thousand-year periods, while the remainder would be progressing on the hundred-million-year scale.

This is exactly the kind of achievement the human race has been making; and this achievement is derived from the development of specialized forms of function within the confines of existing and relatively unchanging anatomy.

The human being is now passing beyond an understanding of himself as a three-dimensional creature moving through some form of time. We must, therefore, accept space-time as the most real way of regarding time. To do so we do not need to learn any new modes of thought or expression or to develop new organs, for we have always been four-dimensional creatures.

Our present rate of advancement may now be seen as the effect of the following principle: *In symmetrical structures—the two mirror-image halves of the brain—the human animal has achieved specialization of function. In anatomical structures that comprise identical cell groups, connections, and supporting tissues there lie the quite separate potentialities of language on the one side, and space-time skills on the other. By this means, the human race is setting itself free from the limitations imposed by having to wait millions of years for new anatomical organs subserving these functions to develop above, beside, or elsewhere in relation to the existing nervous system.*

We must now see ourselves at a critical time of human evolution, at what it is nowadays fashionable to call an "explosive" moment of achievement, of danger and adventure. We are in a mental-technological supernova, wherein an entirely new state of being and possibility has suddenly been thrust upon us. All but a fraction of the human race is now mentally or practically unprepared, and science has not yet begun to study the nature of the new evolutionary force rushing along all about us, already carrying us fast along with it. In the midst of such awesome changes in man, it is habitual for the clinician, the neurologist, and neurosurgeon to press on with diagnosis and treatment, whereas our patients show us every gradation of evolution and dissolution of man's supreme powers, and we may ourselves be obliged to affect these powers by our actions of investigation and treatment. In particular, the neurosurgeon is obliged to act upon a patient mainly because his brain state is altering, and with it his consciousness and personality. Therefore, the neurosurgeon provides—as in the preoperative and postoperative situation—unique material for investigating cerebral function.

We must now see that the slow processes of evolution, which contain many safeguards, seem to be circumvented by forms of specialization of nervous performance directed, mainly without consciousness, towards obviating the need for millions of years of graduality. This statement is the equivalent of a proclamation of entirely new rates of space-time awareness for the human race. The space and time separation is passing from us. As we extend our physical speed and space ranges, new options of time, memory, and age will establish themselves with us.

We must ask ourselves, with deep seriousness, if this theme is not a worthy one for the neurological physician.

Selected Bibliography
of Writings by Walther Riese*

Books

Vincent van Gogh in der Krankheit. Ein Beitrag zum Problem der Beziehung zwischen Kunstwerk und Krankheit. Muenchen, Verlag J. F. Bergmann, 1926.

Das Sinnesleben eines Dichters: Georg Trakl. Stuttgart, Puettmann, 1928.

Der Fall Wiechmann. Zur Psychologie und Soziologie des Familienmordes. Schriften zur Psychologie und Soziologie von Sexualitaet und Verbrechen, herausgegeben von W. Riese und H. Riese. Bd. I., Stuttgart, Puettmann, 1928.

Die Unfallneurose als Problem der Gegenwartsmedizin. In collaboration with others. Stuttgart, Leipzig, Zuerich, Hippokrates-Verlag, 1929.

Die Unfallneurose und das Reichsgericht, mit O. Rothbarth, idem., 1930.

Die Unfallneurose als Problem der Gegenwartsmedizin, Schweiz. Ztschr. f. Unfallmed. u. Berufskrankheiten (Sonderheft traumatische Neurose), 1932.

Das Triebverbrechen. Unmittelbare Ursachen des Sexual- und Affektdelikts, ihre Bedeutung fuer die Zurechnungsfaehigkeit des Taeters, Bern, Verlag Hans Huber, 1933.

L'idée de l'homme dans la neurologie contemporaine, avec A. Réquet, Paris, Alcan, 1938.

La pensée causale en médecine, Presses Universitaires de France, Paris, 1950.

La pensée morale en médecine, premiers principes d'une éthique médicale, Presses Universitaires de France, Paris, 1954.

Principles of Neurology in the Light of History and their Present Use, Nervous and Mental Disease Monographs, New York, 1950; Williams and Wilkins, Baltimore.

---

*Complete bibliography available on request to Dr. Hertha Riese, Rt. 2, Box 397, Glen Allen, Virginia 23060.

228

The Conception of Disease, Its History, Its Versions and Its Nature, Philosophical Library, New York, 1952. Il concetto di malattia (Italian version) translated by Prof. Dr. Giuseppe Ongaro, Episteme editrice, Milano, 1976.

A History of Neurology, M. D. Publications, New York, 1959.

Galen on the Passions and Errors of the Soul. From the Greek by Dr. Paul W. Harkins. Introduction and interpretation by W. Riese, Ohio State University Press, 1963.

La théorie des passions à la lumière de la pensée médicale du dixseptième siècle. Suppl. ad vol. 8, Confinia Psychiatrica, S. Karger, Basel, New York, 1965.

The Legacy of Pinel. An Inquiry into Thought on Mental Alienation, Springer Publishing Co., New York, 1969.

Selected Papers on the History of Aphasia, Neurolinguistics 7, edited by Richard Hoops, Ph.D. and Yvan Lebrun, Ph.D., Swets & Zeitlinger B. V., Amsterdam and Lisse, 1977.

ARTICLES

I.   Principles of Nervous Function; Analyses and Genesis of Symptoms

Voluntary Compensation and Induced Alteration of Tonus (neck reflexes, labyrinth reflexes, etc.): Zeschr. f.d. ges. Neurol. u. Psychiat., 76:367–371, 1922; with K. Goldstein, Klin. Wchnschr., 2:1201–1206; 2:2338–2340, 1923; with Atsushi Iri, 3:187–188, 1924; with K. Goldstein, 4:1201–1204, 1250–1254; and Monatsschr. f. Ohrenh. u. Laryngo-Rhinologie, 58:931–940, 1924.

Clinical and Pathological Studies of Tactile Agnosia: Monatsschr. f. Psychiat. u. Neurol., 62:147–152, 1926; and Arch. f. Psychiat., 82:110–120, 1927.

Neurological and Psychological Studies of Motor Phenomena (facial, speech, and aphasia): Psychol. u. Med., 2:172–183, 1927; Psychol. u. Med., 2:172–183, 1927; Monatsschr. f. Psychiat. u. Neurol., 68:507–514, 1928; and Henschen Anniversary number, J. F. Psychol. u. Neurol., 40:347–355, 1930.

Cortical and Peripheral Disturbances of the Organs of Smell: Handbuch der Neurologie, edited by von O. Bumke and O. Foerster, Berlin, J. Springer, 1935.

Clinical and Neuroanatomical Studies of Rhinal Agenesia: Ztschr. f. d. ges. Neurol. u. Psychiat., 69:303–317, 1921; with K. Goldstein, J. F. Psychol. u. Neurol., 32:291–311, 1925-26; and Deutsche Ztschr. f. Nervenh., 89:37–44, 1926.

II.   Comparative Neurology and Pathology

On Aquatic Mammals: Anat. Anz., 57:487–494, 1923–24; Ztschr. f. d. ges. Neurol. u. Psychiat., 90:591–598, 1924; J. F. Psychol. u. Neurol., 31:275–280, 1924-25; 32:21–28, 1925; 32:281–290, 1925-26; 34:

194–201, 1926; 33:84–96, 1927; Anat. Anz., 65:225–260, 1928; and Proc. Kon. Ned. Akad. van Wetenschappen, 39:97–109, 1936.

The Brain and Its Function in Newborn Mammals and Problems of Cortical Evolution: (1) *Bear:* Compt. rend. Academie des Sciences, 206: 1834–1837, 1938; Bull. du Museum National d'Histoire Naturelle, t.X. No. 6, 1938; Proc. Kon. Med. Akad. van Wetenschappen, 42:208–214, 1939; Rev. gen. des Sciences, 50:2–3, 1939; Compt. rend. Academie des Sciences, 208:465–468, 1939; Rev. canad. de biol., 1:157–170, 1942. (2) *Marsupial:* with G. E. Smyth, Proc. Kon. Med. Akad. van Wetenschappen, 43:2–8, 1940; Le Naturaliste Canadien, 70:139–144, 1943; J. of Mammalogy, 26:148–153, 1945; and 29:150–155, 1948.

III. Neuroanatomy and Neuropathology

The Human Brain in Old Age: J. Neuropath. and Exper. Neurol., 5:160–164, 1946; Rev. neurol., 81:227–229, 1949; J. Exper. Neurol. and Neuropath., 12:92–93, 1953; J. Comp. Neurol., 100:525–568, 1954.

Brains of Prominent Scholars in Advanced Age: J. Exper. Neurol. and Neuropath., 12:92–93, 1953; J. Comp. Neurol., 100:525–568, 1954.

Tumor Symptomatology Manifested in Terms of Age: Rev. neurol., 81: 227–229, 1949; 85:72–73 and 400–401, 1951; With G. S. Fultz, Am. J. Psychiat., 106:206–211, 1949; Revue Neurol., 94:88–89, 1956.

Momentum of Growth: Confinia neurol., 9:64–79, 1949; Rev. neurol., 84: 192–193, 1951; J. Nerv. and Ment. Dis., 131:291–301, 1960; Schweiz. Arch. f. Neurol. Neurochir. u. Psychiat., 84:172–179, 1959.

Diaschisis: Internat'l. Rec. of Med., 171:73–82, 1958; L'Encephale, 37:183–194, 1946–47.

Changing Concepts of Localization and Dynamics of Brain Lesions: Hyg. Ment., 31:105–136, 1936; Hyg. ment., 31:137–158, 1936; with E. C. Hoff, J. Hist. Med. and Allied Sc., 1:50–71, 1950; Arch. f. Neurol., Neurochir., u. Psychiat., 88:299–314, 1961; Clio Medica, 2:189–230, 1967.

Lateral Dominance: Its Nature and Historical Versions: Clio Medica, 5:319–326, 1970.

Aphasia: Psychol. u. Med., 2:172–183, 1927; Monatsschr. f. Psychiat. u. Neurol., 68:507–514, 1928; with A. Merzbach, Ztschr. f. Voelkerpsychol., u. Soziol., 4:44–53, 1928; Confinia neurol., 9:64–79, 216–225, 1949; Rev. neurol., 92:146–147, 1955; J. Nerv. and Ment. Dis., 123:18–22, 1956; L'Encephale, 4:437–467, 1957; J. Nerv. and Ment. Dis., 128:302–308, 1959; Rev. neurol., 100:488–489, 1959; J. Nerv. and Ment. Dis., 138:293–295, 1964.

Sub-Cortical Affections: Confinia neurol., 9:216–225, 1949.

IV. Neuropathology of Mental Disorders

Rev. neurol., 81:785–787, 1949; Am. J. Psychiat., 106:206–211, 1949; Rev. neurol., 82:137–139, 1950; C. and O. Vogt Anniversary number, Monatsschr. f. Psychiat. u. Nervenkrankheiten, 1950.

V. History and Philosophy of Medicine

Archives suisses de neurol. et de psychiat., 44:313–319, 1939; J. Nerv.
and Ment. Dis., 96:296–312, 1942; 98:255–266, 1943; 100:263–274,
1944; Bull. Hist. Med., 23:546–533, 1949; Arch. suisses de neurol.
et de psychiat., 41:410–422, 1938; J. Nerv. and Ment. Dis., 131:291–
301, 1960; J. Nerv. and Ment. Dis., 132:469–484, 1961; (Galen)
Revue Philosophique de la France et de l'Etranger, Paris, 153: 331–
346, 1963; (Maimonide) Rev. Hist. Med. Hebraique, no. 54, pp. 149–
153, 1961; (Descartes) Med. Hist., 10:237–244, 1966; (Kant) Rev.
philo. no. 3, pp. 327–333, July 1965; (Existentialism) J. of Exis., No.
21, 6:89–97, 1965; (Causal Thought) Episteme, No. 1, pp. 3–16,
1967; Episteme, No. 2, pp. 111-120, 1968; Episteme, No. 2, pp. 135–
140, 1972.

VI. Analytical and Experimental Thought and Method

Bull. Hist. Med., 14:281–294, 1943; (Claude Bernard) Acta Biotheoretica,
12:187–194, 1958; Schweiz. Ztschr. f. Psychol. u. ihre Anwend., 19:
321–324, 1960; Studies in Romanticism, The Graduate School, Boston
University, 2 (1): 11–22, 1962; (Condillac and Pinel) Revue Phil.
pp. 321–336, 1968; (Pinel) L'Evolution Psych. No. 2, pp. 407–413,
1966; (Bacon and Claude Bernard) Episteme, No. 2, 167–171, 1967;
Recherches Psycho-Phar., pp. 78–91, P.U.F., Paris, 1967; (Aristotle to
Claude Bernard) Episteme, No. 2, pp. 111-120, 1968; Bull. de l'Acad.
Nat. de Med., 3e serie, t. 152, pp. 145–149, 1968; Bull. de l'Acad.
Nationale de Med., 3e serie, t. 152, pp. 560–563, 1968; (Moreau de
Tours) Episteme, No. 3, pp. 210–213, 1969; Bull. de l'Acad. Na-
tionale de Med., t. 154, pp. 28–29, 1970.

VII. Precursors of Present-Day Medicine

(Claude Bernard) Bull. Hist. Med., 14:281–294, 1943; Bull. Hist. Med.,
18:465–512, 1945; (Goldstein) Schweiz. Arch. f. Neurol., u. Psychiat.,
62:1–10, 1948; Bull. Hist. Med., 23:111–136, 1949; (Goethe) Bull.
Hist. Med., 23:546–553, 1949; (Hughlings Jackson) J. Nerv. and Ment.
Dis., 120:330–337, 1954; with W. Gooddy, Bull. Hist. Med., 29:230–
238, 1955; J. Nerv. and Ment. Dis., 124:125–134, 1956; Sci. and
Psychoanal., Grune & Stratton, New York, pp. 29–72, 1958; J. Nerv.
and Ment. Dis., 127:287–307, 1958; (Muller) with G. E. Arrington,
Am. J. of Ophth., 47:185–186, 1959; Internat'l. Rec. of Med., 173:
7–19, 1960; Rev. Philosophique de la Fr. et de l'Etranger, 150:145–
162, 1960; (Burrow) Suppl. to vol. 11, 5–36, Acta Psychother. and
Psychosomatica, 1963; Schweiz. Arch. f. Neurol., Neurochir., u. Psychiat., 88:299–314, 1961; (Muller) with G. E. Arrington, Bull. Hist.
Med., 37:179–183, 1963; (Galen) Bull. N.Y. Acad. of Med., 44:778–
791, 1968; Rev. Philosophique, pp. 321–336, 1968; (Pinel) Soc.
Moreau de Tours Ann. Ther. Psychiat., 4, 130–148, 1969; Episteme,
No. 2, pp. 247–251, 1972.

VIII.   Forensic, Sociopsychiatric, and Socioneurological Studies

Acta Psychiat. et neurol., 3:153–164, 1928; Hippokrates, 1:87–95, 1928; Monatsschr. f. Kriminalpsychol. u. Strafrechtsreform, 20:428–433, 1929; Muenchen. med. Wchnschr., 76:928–929, 1929; Internat. Ztschr. f. Sozialversicherung, 1929; Allg. aerztl. Ztschr. f. Psychotherap. u. psych. Hyg., 1:509–519, 1928; Die Justiz, 4:603–618, 618–621, 1928–29; Ztschr. f. Psychotherap. u. psych. Hyg., 2:741–752, 1929; Deutsche med. Wchnschr., 55:1244–1246, 1929; Der Nervenarzt, 3:65–68, 1930; Schweiz. Arch. f. Neurol. u. Psychiat., 25:300–305, 1930; Die Justiz, 7:103–117, 1931; Monatsschr. f. Kriminalpsychol. u. Strafrechtsreform, 22:730–734, 1931; Allg. Ztschr. f. Psychiat., 98: 417–422, 1932; Aertzl. Sachverst. Ztg., 38:225–228, 1932; Schweiz. Arch. f. Neurol. u. Psychiat., 32:95–104, 215–244, 1933; Ztschr. f. d. ges. gerichtliche Med., 1933; Schweiz. Arch. f. Neurol. u. Psychiat., 34: 159–164, 1934; L'evolution psychiatrique, 4:81–87, 1935; Arch. suisses de neurol. et de psychiat., 41:410–422, 1938.

IX.   Psychopathology of Famous Authors, Poets and Painters

(Kleist) Allg. Ztschr. f. Psychiat., 96:270–312, 1932; (Van Gogh) CIBA-Symposium, vol. VI:198–205, 1958 (also in German, French, Dutch, Spanish, and Italian languages); (Goya) Episteme, 1965.

X.   Articles in Honor of, or Concerning, Prominent Authors

(Goldstein) The Reach of Mind: Essays in Memory of Kurt Goldstein, ed. Marianne L. Simmel, Springer Publishing Co., New York, pp. 245–250, 1968; Historic Derivations of Modern Psychiatry, ed. Iago Galdston, M.D., McGraw-Hill, New York, pp. 75–137, 1967; Schweiz. Arch. f. Neurol. u. Psychiat., 62:1–10, 1948; (Pagel) Sci., Med. and Society in the Renaissance, Sci. Hist. Pub., New York, pp. 163–165, 1972.

XI.   Contributions to Encyclopedias and Collective Works

Histoire Universelle de la Med. (Madrid) vol. VI, pp. 235–240, 1974; Essays to Honor Walter Pagel, ed. Allen C. Debus, Univ. of Chicago, 1975; (A. Strumpell) The Founders of Neurology, ed. W. Haymaker and K. Baer, Army Med. Lib., Wash., D.C., Thomas, Springfield, Ill., 1951; Problems of Dynamic Neurology, ed. Prof. Dr. L. Halpern, Hadassah Med. Org. and Hebrew Univ., Jerusalem, Israel, pp. 1–29, 1963; (Muller) Founders of Neurology, ed. W. Haymaker and F. Schiller, Univ. of Cal., 1953 and 1970.

DATE DUE

GAYLORD			PRINTED IN U.S.A.